thank you mummy for all
the lovely me
cook for me

GW00727905

SMART BABY
COOKBOOK

BOOST YOUR BABY'S IMMUNITY
AND BRAIN DEVELOPMENT

LAUREN CHENEY

MURDOCH BOOKS
SYDNEY · LONDON

John Travers

— x x x —

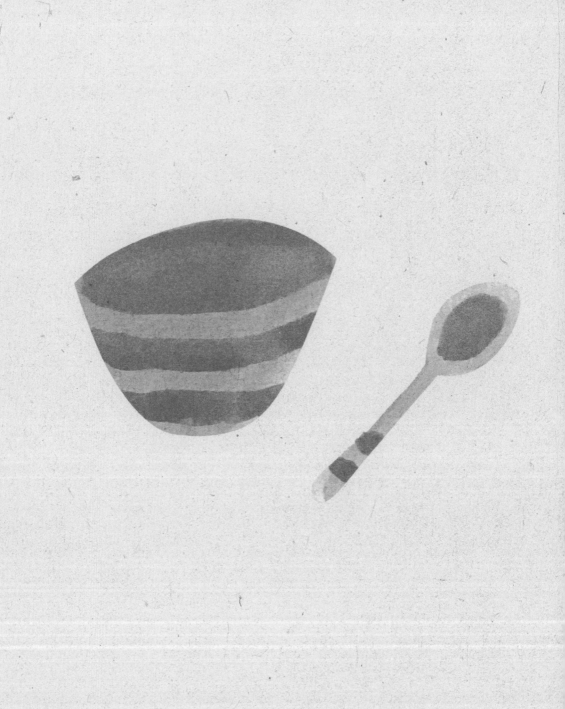

FOREWORD

We all want the absolute best for our children. From the moment they are born we strive to provide them with the best care and comfort in the hope that they will grow up to be healthy, loving, well-adjusted adults who make the most of their unique talents and abilities. We want them to reach their full potential.

As a paediatrician and mother of two, I know the pathway to health, optimal brain function and a robust immune system lies in consuming a nutritious diet that supplies all the valuable nutrients, right from the first baby foods. What your child is fed in the first three years of life has an enormous impact. While 'nature' and genes are certainly the basis for some of your child's development, 'nurture' is most definitely responsible for a significant portion. It is crucial for parents to understand that they can dramatically influence their child's cognitive function and health by simply getting diet right in those important first three years.

This is where the *Smart Baby Cookbook* can help. It provides parents with the information they need to make informed decisions when weaning their babies. In my line of work I often come across parents who are nervous about the weaning process or do not have the appropriate knowledge to make the best food choices. In many cases they are using outdated information that has been gleaned from relatives or other parents.

Educating parents about the best way to feed their children should be given high priority in prenatal visits and definitely be first on the agenda during postnatal visits. This book fills a gap by providing dietary advice and recipes that are aimed at giving children the best chance to reach their potential.

I regularly witness the benefits of proper nutrition, seeing children who have fewer allergies, fewer behavioural problems, fewer chronic illnesses and fewer digestive issues. I highly recommend this book to anyone who is invested in helping their child towards a healthy life.

Dr Natalia Vollrath-Hale
Paediatrician, MD, FRACP

CONTENTS

ABOUT THE AUTHOR

I dedicate this book to the love of my life: my son, Oscar.

I am a mum on a mission, stay-at-home chef, domestically challenged housewife and functioning coffee addict, determined to better the health outcomes of the next generation, one 'aeroplane spoon' at a time.

Most days you will find me in the kitchen, wrestling the last of the eggs from my toddler, who loves to get his hands dirty cooking up a storm but has not yet mastered the art of keeping a clean kitchen.

My love of cooking comes from evenings spent as a child, watching my father turn our dinners into a magical experience. His love of creating Mediterranean meals and serving them with matching music was a delight for the whole family. It started a passion in me that was to fuel my love of cooking for years to come.

Fast forward to the day I became a mother and what followed was the catalyst to creating the *Smart Baby Cookbook*. Oscar was born with an extremely rare, life-threatening and lifelong immune disorder called Pulmonary Lymphangiectasia. By the time of his birth, five weeks early, Oscar had already undergone three lung operations in utero. I was advised that he had a very vulnerable immune system and might be developmentally affected.

I was determined to give Oscar the best chance of leading a healthy and happy life, especially as he had fought so hard for it. I made it my mission to talk to as many health professionals as possible. I also put my nutritional knowledge and chef experience to use, researching ingredients and developing meals that would naturally boost his immunity and development.

My purpose was twofold: I wanted to cook foods that not only turned Oscar into the next super-healthy Einstein, but also encouraged him to be a little 'foodie' who would enjoy family meals. Like so many parents of small children, I simply didn't have the energy or brain power to cook food that was suitable for him and then create an entirely new meal for my husband and me. I knew there had to be a better way.

With evidence-based science proving that good digestive health is linked to overall health, from the gut to the brain, we have the potential to optimise immunity and brain development right from our child's very first foods. The search for nutritious recipes led me to research smart foods – ingredients that benefit and promote gut health. I was particularly interested in the field of neuroscience and how specific foods support and boost brain function and development. Society is becoming more health conscious: it only makes sense that we try our hardest to feed our children the best foods. We have the potential to write a blueprint that could help prevent certain diseases and even maximise intelligence.

I was urged to share my recipes and research when the doctors were amazed at Oscar's increased immunity levels and cognitive development. I spent two years researching and collaborating with child health experts to help other families set their children on the path to good health from their earliest years.

It is my hope that the *Smart Baby Cookbook* will be used as a resource by time-poor parents, who want to ensure that their family receives all the benefits of a super-nutritious, flavoursome meal without having to cook separately for adults and children, or serve dulled-down baby food.

For me, food means family. I believe that shared meals not only empower our children to develop a love of healthy food and help to create adventurous eaters, but also deliver a wonderful bonding moment and a little meal-time magic. Happy cooking everyone.

smartlittlefoodie.com.au

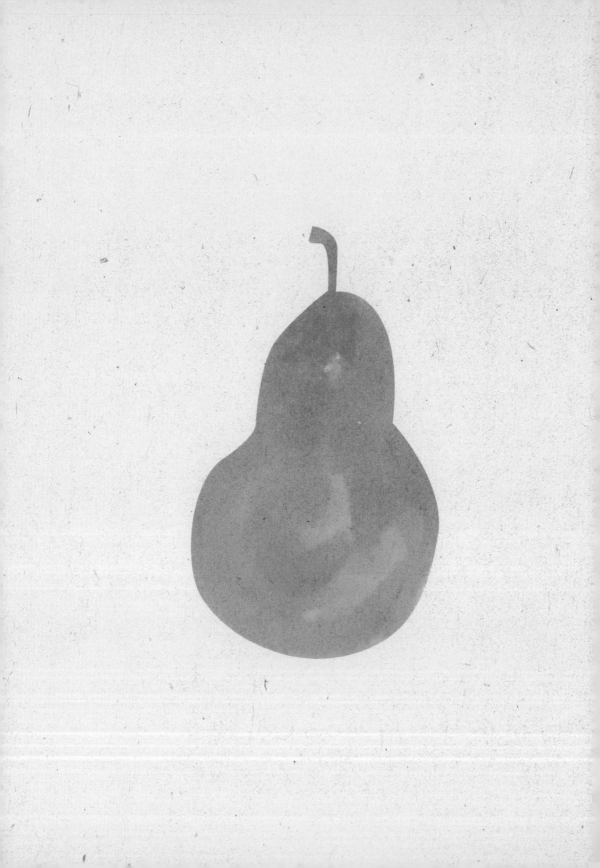

INTRODUCTION

Take away the rose-tinted glasses of early parenthood, the in-laws whose children have been perfect eaters since day one, the friends with strategically posed Facebook photos of baby Archie/Amber enjoying 'Purea di pollo e verdure' (aka puréed chicken and vegetables) and you will find a little-mentioned truth, the seedy underbelly of starting solids.

Here's a hint of what lies ahead – tantrums, thousands of clothing changes, endless laundry, snorting of unknown substances, 120-decibel screaming, food refusal, toxic poo, grabbing of breasts and constant whining for a drink. No, it's not the Rolling Stones, it's worse... It's your child and at first they can't get no satisfaction when the breast is away and vegetables are the meal of the day.

We are hard-wired to pacify our child, but this new stage means getting a little tough, a little inventive and a whole lot tenacious. Time to put on your hard hat, tighten the heart strings and step up to the dinner plate. When times are tough and you're wearing puréed pumpkin on your head, just remember, you're in it for the long haul and what you do now paves the way for your child's future physical and cognitive health.

Unique to the market, the *Smart Baby Cookbook* includes only recipes that aim to increase baby's immunity and brain development. But this is more than just a powerhouse cookbook: it is a survival guide designed to help take your mini-me from first bite to finger food and beyond with a minimum of fuss and a maximum of good health.

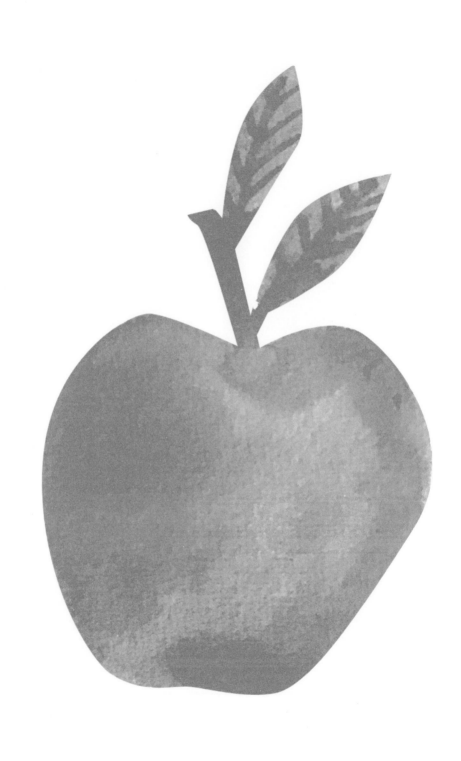

HELP!
I'M
FREAKING
OUT!

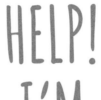

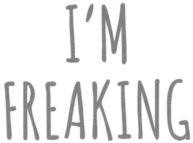

CHAPTER 1

WHEN TO START SOLIDS

Until your baby turns one breastmilk or formula is still their most important food source. If you start baby on solids too early their digestive system and kidneys will not be fully adjusted to the change of nutrition.

On the other hand, introducing your baby to solids too late might interfere with their iron requirements. When a baby reaches six months of age their iron stores start to deplete and they require iron-rich foods to maintain them. There is also some evidence that delaying the introduction of solid food could also delay basic chewing skills, which can affect speech development.

Meanwhile, you're probably tired of being at baby's mercy when it comes to scheduling your own activities around feeding times; and your partner is wondering when he's ever going to get another look at the sexy little negligée that started all of this. So when can you call the grandparents and schedule your next date night? How do you know when your baby is ready to start eating solid food?

Every baby is different, but generally they will be ready to start solid food at around four to six months. At this time most will easily accept new flavours and textures. However, every baby is an individual and they all develop at different rates, so it's important to recognise signs that might indicate your baby is ready.

IS YOUR BABY READY FOR SOLIDS?
ANSWER THESE QUESTIONS...

Are they over 18? Only kidding! We all know that's the age they go back to drinking. Sigh. Parenthood is an endless cycle – by the time you've got it all down pat, they'll be feeding you the puréed vegetables. Anyway, back to those questions...

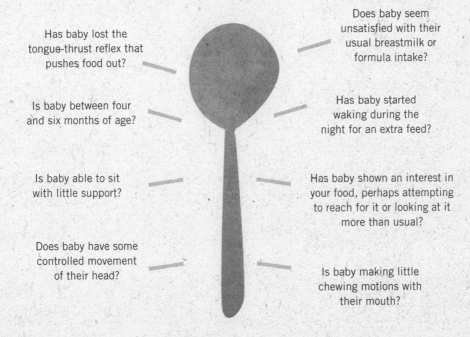

Has baby lost the tongue-thrust reflex that pushes food out?

Is baby between four and six months of age?

Is baby able to sit with little support?

Does baby have some controlled movement of their head?

Does baby seem unsatisfied with their usual breastmilk or formula intake?

Has baby started waking during the night for an extra feed?

Has baby shown an interest in your food, perhaps attempting to reach for it or looking at it more than usual?

Is baby making little chewing motions with their mouth?

If you answered 'yes' to most of these, it's probably a good time to start feeding your baby some solid food.

FOOD ALLERGENS

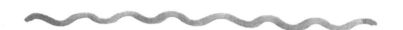

And so now you have the next important parenting decision: which foods to introduce first and which are considered unsafe. Take the introduction of peanut-based foods, for example. You might be so worried that you find yourself sitting in a hospital car park with 37 other mums and babies, all nervously clutching jars of peanut butter and spoons, with EpiPens (epinephrine autoinjectors) at the ready in case of allergic reaction.

We don't advise going that far – it pays to remember that the incidence of food allergy in babies is relatively small. However, if there is a family history or risk of allergy then it is advisable to discuss any concerns with your doctor and have your baby tested before starting solids.

Under old guidelines, weaning used to be a complicated task and parents were instructed to introduce foods in a special order. However, the latest research states that there is no need for this and, with the exception of a few foods (see page 17), you can decide for yourself what foods you would like to feed your baby and in what order. We advise giving baby a wholefoods diet with a focus on prebiotic and probiotic foods (see page 23).

With regard to high-allergen foods, current advice is to introduce them at around the six-month mark. It is thought that introducing allergens along with other foods affords better protection against developing allergies. In fact, there is increasing evidence that delaying the introduction of certain foods might increase the risk of developing a food allergy.

The current Australasian Society of Clinical Immunology and Allergy (ASCIA) guidelines are that all infants should be given allergenic foods, including peanut butter, cooked egg, dairy and wheat products, in the first year of life. This includes infants who are at high risk of allergy. For example, there is moderate evidence that introducing cooked egg (raw egg is not recommended) into an

infant's diet before eight months of age can reduce the risk
of developing an egg allergy, even if there is a family history.

There is no need to wait three to five days between offering
different foods. However, when offering a food that is known to
cause allergies, it is advisable to wait 24–48 hours after each
offering so you can monitor for an allergic reaction or intolerance.

Although allergic reactions usually occur from a few minutes to
an hour after consuming a food for the first time, it is also possible
to have an allergic reaction only after the second or third time.

In rare cases anaphylaxis can occur: baby might appear floppy,
droopy, drowsy or pale, or have facial swelling and breathing
difficulties. If any of these occur call an ambulance immediately.
An allergic reaction can also present as hives, itchiness, red skin,
vomiting, coughing, wheezing and bowel issues.

These are the foods that most commonly cause reactions:

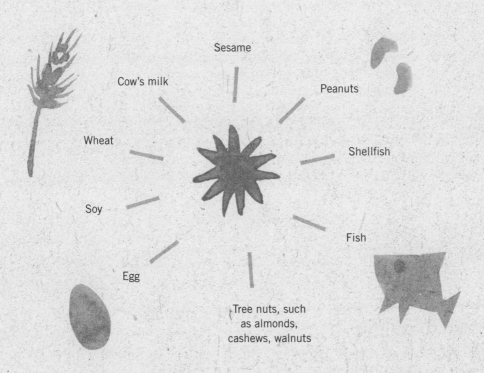

Sesame

Cow's milk

Peanuts

Wheat

Shellfish

Soy

Fish

Egg

Tree nuts, such
as almonds,
cashews, walnuts

GOING NUTS

Although delaying the introduction of foods does not reduce the incidence of food allergy, that doesn't mean you should hand Junior a bag of walnuts and cross your fingers. Whole and chopped nuts are not suitable for children under the age of five because they pose a risk of choking.

However, nuts are a valuable source of 'good' fats (which protect brain health in infants) so, to ensure bub is not missing out on this valuable food, grind the nuts down and mix them into purées and finger foods. Many health-food stores sell ready-made nut meal, which makes a great addition to breakfast.

The World Health Organization advocates introducing nuts to infants from six months on. A study conducted in 2008 [note 1, page 175] concluded that waiting to introduce nuts can prove counterproductive: early consumption of nuts seems to be related to a lower risk of allergies. ASCIA also states that a regular peanut intake before 12 months of age can help reduce the risk of developing peanut allergy.

If you are at all concerned, then talk to your doctor before introducing commonly allergenic foods.

WHAT TO DRINK

Babies do not generally require water when they are beginning solids, as most of their needs are still being met by breastmilk or formula; however, by the time they are eight or nine months old, they should be offered water at every meal to assist the kidneys and prevent constipation. A spill-proof cup of cooled boiled water will give baby a chance to practise using a cup and also get them used to the taste.

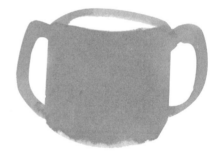

FOOD & DRINKS TO AVOID

COW'S MILK

Not recommended as baby's main milk supply because it can interfere with iron requirements. However, cow's milk can be used on cereal and in cooking.

FRUIT JUICE & SWEETENED DRINKS

Offer no nutritional benefit to babies under 12 months of age.

LOW-FAT DAIRY

Not recommended for children under two years of age.

HONEY

Might contain botulinum spores. Not recommended for children under 12 months of age.

WHOLE PEANUTS & SMALL, HARD, ROUND FOODS

Might be a choking hazard. Even grapes should be cut into pieces or mashed.

RAW, UNDERCOOKED & FERMENTED MEATS

Risk of salmonella poisoning.

SALT

Do not add salt to food: developing kidneys might be affected. Check labels of ready-made food for sodium levels.

FISH HIGH IN MERCURY

Sea perch, catfish, flake, marlin and swordfish are best avoided.

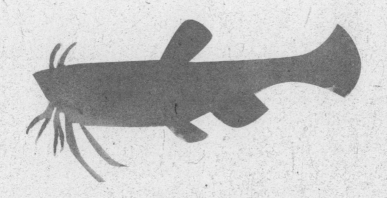

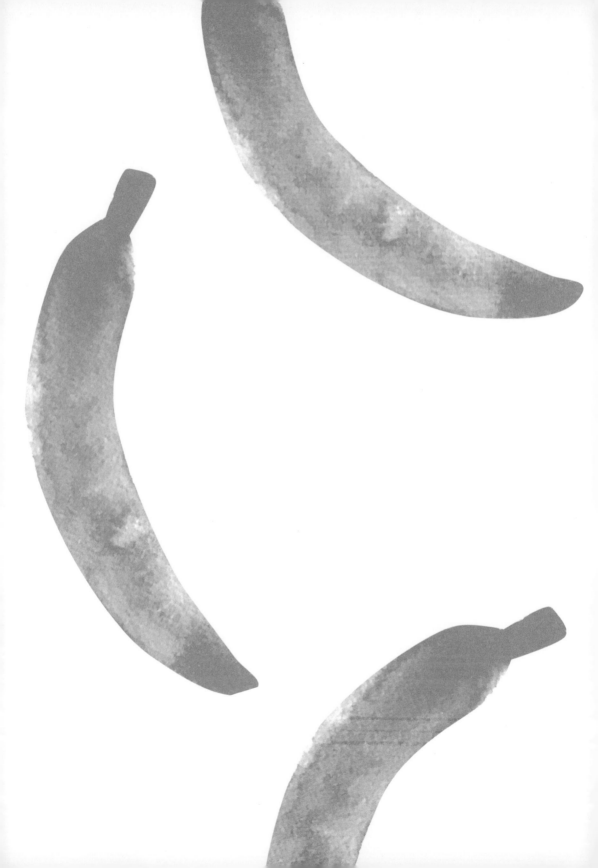

SMART FOODS

CHAPTER 2

WHAT ARE SMART FOODS?

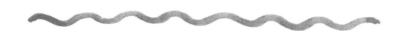

This book aims to provide recipes that include specific wholefoods for optimal nutritional balance and PROTECTIVE and PREVENTATIVE nutrition.

SMART FOODS:

Strengthen the immune system

Maximise optimal nutrient uptake

Aid cognitive development

Reinforce good gut health

Turn on 'good gene' expression

Perhaps the most important thing you can learn is how significant the first three years of life are when it comes to laying the groundwork for baby's health now and in the future. Nutrition is often considered the single greatest environmental influence during infancy. It can have long-term effects on health, intelligence, ability and predisposition to disease.

From birth, cells are growing and dividing and neural pathways are being formed. These processes are highly sensitive to and affected by what goes into the body. The nutrients available to each cell as it grows and divides have a direct impact on how efficiently it functions, now and in the future.

About half the food an infant consumes goes towards nourishing and sustaining brain activity, so you can begin to understand why it is so important to make quality food choices on your baby's behalf. You are switching on your baby's body and brain and keeping them running smoothly when you make smart food choices.

Smart foods promote good health through protective and preventative nutrition. Adhering to a nutritionally balanced diet that incorporates wholefoods during a baby's formative years and beyond is critical for brain development. It will also give your child the best chance of living a disease-free life.

Nutrient deficiencies affect cell production and communication, and a lack of nutrients, such as iron and iodine, can also impair cognitive and motor development. In addition, our Western diet, with its refining, processing, preserving and sterilising of foods, has removed much of the microbiota and fibre that is essential for good digestive health.

This is where good nutrition from an early age can help.

FEEDING THE BRAIN

The brain reaches a whopping 80 per cent of its adult weight during the first two years of life. That's a lot of grey matter! So, in essence, what we feed our children in the first few years really does have an impact on their brain power.

Child health researcher Dr Anett Nyaradi has conducted several long-term studies about the effect of food on brain function. She says that 'a good diet may be especially beneficial in the first year of life'. In her studies [note 2], which began in 1989, she recorded the dietary intake of a cohort of children, then compared them to academic results in standardised testing in primary school and cognitive testing as teenagers. The results showed that those children who were breastfed and then consumed a more nutritious diet in their early years demonstrated better outcomes. The conclusion was that what a child ate during the first years of life is likely to have a significant effect on brain development and therefore cognitive performance in later life.

Other studies [notes 3; 4; 5] found that children who consumed higher amounts of fruit, vegetables and home-cooked food during infancy had higher IQ scores at four years of age; and that there are negative associations between the consumption of ready-made baby foods at early ages and IQ scores at eight years old.

A BRAIN BLUEPRINT

Overwhelmed by all this information and responsibility? Don't be. This book is all about smart foods that support digestive health, enhance brain function, optimise nutrient balance, prevent inflammation and boost the immune system.

Most parents don't have the time to wade through scientific literature to figure out how to incorporate the latest beneficial findings into their family's daily nutrition, so we've created an easy-to-follow blueprint. It translates the latest exciting findings about infant nutrition into an action plan. During early childhood the machinery of the brain is particularly sensitive to environmental factors such as nutrition and there is a growing body of paediatric research that supports the benefits of the Mediterranean diet for children. For example, children who more closely followed the principles of a Mediterranean diet had a lower risk of obesity.

Simply put, the Mediterranean diet is wholefood nutrition. It is loaded with fibre, vitamins, minerals, antioxidants and phytochemicals. The food is fresh, balanced and eaten seasonally. This is more than a diet; it is a way of life and one that is centred on family. From their very first foods, babies share flavoursome family meals and children develop a love and appreciation of nutritious food that lasts a lifetime.

With a focus on vegetables, fruits, legumes, nuts, seeds, whole grains, fish, poultry, grass-fed meats, dairy, 'good fats', herbs and spices, this book uses the principles of the Mediterranean diet. People who adhere to this traditional diet have been identified as living long lives and having a lower occurrence of disease. Consistently following a Mediterranean diet is thought to provide some protection from nearly all our most serious conditions, including cancer, cardiovascular disease, Alzheimer's and diabetes.

Our recipes advocate wholefoods that contain the macronutrients and micronutrients that are missing in refined and processed foods. Our well-balanced, tasty recipes can also help to prevent your baby becoming a fussy eater. Since babies learn through exploration of texture, taste, smell and appearance, we have deliberately created colourful and tactile recipes that help stimulate those rapidly growing neural pathways, while also building a robust microbiome.

PROBIOTICS & PREBIOTICS

Probiotics are 'good' bacteria that help control the growth of harmful bacteria, and prebiotics are food that feed and nourish the 'good' bacteria. Both are equally important for a healthy digestive system. Helping to improve the 'good-to-bad' bacteria ratio has been shown to have a direct correlation to overall health. To help strengthen your little one's microbiome, try to include the following foods in their regular diet...

Probiotics: Natural yoghurt with live cultures.

Prebiotics: Garlic; Onion; Asparagus; Leek; Jerusalem artichokes; Bananas; Legumes; Oatmeal; Apple peel.

SPICE IT UP

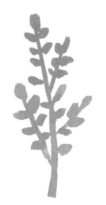

Believe it or not, baby food can be packed with flavour. It's all in the herbs and spices you add to the main ingredients. Not convinced baby will take to a mildly spiced dish? Well, consider this: babies are exposed to herbs and spices in the womb and, if you are breastfeeding, your baby is also getting a taste for the flavours of herbs and spices through your breastmilk.

Babies throughout the world readily take to herbs and spices. An Indian child does not suddenly develop a taste for the aromatic curries of their culture unless they have been exposed to them as a baby. It is no different with your baby. Offering food flavoured with herbs and spices helps foster a taste for non-bland foods and creates adventurous eaters who will choose good food over the dreaded 'chicken nuggets and chips' on many children's menus. Don't wait until your child is a toddler before you introduce them: it might be too late by then. If you start baby young enough, you might find they aren't drawn to sugary or salty foods so much when they are older. Besides adding flavour, herbs and spices offer

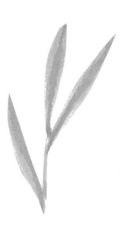

health benefits of their own. The following have been shown to reduce inflammation and benefit the brain: turmeric, ginger, garlic, oregano, thyme, rosemary, onion, sage, parsley, nutmeg, basil, curry, cinnamon, cumin and cloves.

SALT

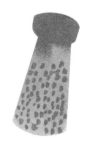

Avoid adding salt to baby's food or cooking with salt. If you're using our 2-in-1 recipes and you like a bit of salt in your meal, add it to your own dish after serving. A baby's kidneys and digestive system are still developing and cannot cope with too much salt. Many sauces and tinned foods contain added salt so become aware of hidden salts by reading labels and looking at the sodium content. Choose 'no added salt' varieties where possible.

FATS

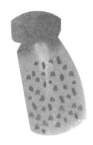

There is no need to give infants low-fat versions of dairy products such as yoghurt and cheese. Babies require full-fat foods with all the vitamins they contain to meet their energy needs. For a long time people were led to believe that all fat was bad for you. Unfortunately this misconception still rings true with a lot of people, but it simply is not. When you consider the fact that more than half the human brain is composed of fat, it makes sense that fats help the brain to function correctly and should be an essential part of our diet; they offer fuel and protection for our brain. It is essential that babies receive adequate amounts of 'good' fats in their diet, in particular fats containing omega–3.

SALMON is nutrient dense and full of protein, vitamins and minerals as well as a great source of omega–3.

YOGHURT contains probiotics important for gut health, which has a direct link to brain health.

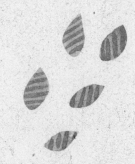

SOURCES OF 'GOOD' FATS

NUTS contain vitamin E. Almonds, pecans and walnuts are best as they can have a protective effect on the brain. A handful a day is enough.

EGGS can promote good memory and assist in overall brain function. They contain vitamins B12, B2, A, B5, selenium and choline, all of which are great for brain and body.

AVOCADO is good for your heart, promotes healthy blood flow, helps lower cholesterol and assists in the control of blood pressure. It is a good source of folate and vitamins C, K, B5, B6 and E and is high in fibre.

OLIVE OIL contains beneficial fatty acids and vitamins K and E, which can have a protective effect on the brain, assist memory and help prevent dementia. Buy extra virgin olive oil – this is the best for you and does not contain 'mixer' oils.

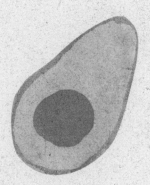

THE SMART TWENTY

To give your child the best start in life, we would like you to meet the Smart Twenty. With a focus on foods that support digestive and cognitive health, giving your baby's brain and body the best start in life is easy when you include a well-balanced variety of wholefoods in their diet.

1 ROOT VEGETABLES

Root vegetables are an excellent source of fibre and phytonutrients. Their high levels of antioxidants help take care of your overall health. From mash to dips and Roast Vegetable Chips (page 50) there are so many ways to serve them, so make sure you are offering your little one a wide variety. Apart from the increased nutritional benefit, variety will help build familiarity; this is key in helping to increase taste preference and prevent future fussiness.

2 CHICKPEAS (GARBANZO BEANS)

Chickpeas are praised for their high fibre content and are a staple of the Mediterranean diet. The insoluble fibre in chickpeas helps treat and prevent constipation, perfect for helping bub stay regular. These little powerhouses also have a high choline content, which aids sleep, muscle movement, learning and memory. High in vitamins and minerals, chickpeas are associated with possible health benefits from helping to prevent diabetes, inflammation and cancer, to protecting the heart, blood pressure and bone health. Hummus is a fantastic way to start your mini-me off on the wonderful health benefits that chickpeas can deliver.

3 FISH

Omega–3 fats accumulate in the brain during foetal development. The amount of omega–3 docosahexaenoic acid (DHA) has been closely tied to cognitive performance in infancy and childhood. It is recommended that children eat fish twice a week to receive the amount of omega–3 their developing brains need. Salmon and sardines are very rich sources of DHA and can be made into anything from fish fingers to salmon egg rolls and sardine sandwiches.

4 TURMERIC

Researchers believe that the antioxidant and anti-inflammatory properties of the curcumin in turmeric might be strong enough to boost brain function. Don't be scared to start using turmeric as soon as your child starts eating solid food.

You can easily build turmeric into many meals by mixing it into vegetable purées and mashes, meat rubs and mild curries (such as Tiny tots' turmeric chicken, page 100).

5 CELERY

Luteolin, found in celery, is a plant compound with anti-inflammatory properties. Celery also has antimicrobial properties to help fight infections.

6 BROCCOLI

Broccoli is a great source of vitamin K, which enhances cognitive function and memory. Packing numerous nutrients, broccoli decreases the risk of diabetes, heart disease and cancer. Yes, these little trees are notorious for being rejected by our small offspring, but, with so many health benefits, the earlier you incorporate broccoli into your child's diet, the better.

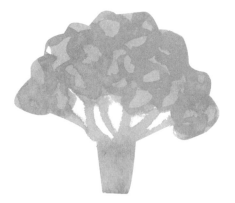

7 EGGS

Eggs are powerhouses of nutrition, containing a little bit of almost every nutrient we require. They also contain choline, which is particularly important for brain and nervous system function. Eggs are an important food to feed your baby, but you must ensure they are thoroughly cooked to avoid any risk of salmonella poisoning.

8 WALNUTS

These nuts don't just look like tiny brains, they contain alpha-Linolenic acid (ALA), which promotes blood flow, helping the brain to receive optimal levels of oxygen. Try to build walnuts into your child's daily diet by adding ground nuts to purées, smoothies, cereals, gratins, pasta and pesto. Remember, whole or chopped nuts pose a choking risk. Walnuts should be stored in an airtight container in your refrigerator to prevent the 'good' fats being damaged.

9 BEANS & LENTILS

Offering a great source of protein, vitamins and minerals, beans feature heavily in the Mediterranean diet. The soluble and insoluble fibre they contain both work to keep the digestive system running smoothly. Soft beans are a great finger food option.

10 RED MEAT

Red meat is still one of the best ways to get a fix of iron and vitamin B12, both essential for a healthy brain. Because a baby's natural iron stores start to deplete as they reduce their breastmilk or formula intake, it is crucial that they are fed iron-rich foods. Red meat is also an important source of zinc, which helps the immune system function properly, while the protein in meat helps build bones and muscles. Check out our starter meat purées on pages 79–80.

11 BLUEBERRIES (& OTHER BERRIES)

Berries are the bomb! They boost immunity, protect your heart and might even help prevent the development of certain cancers. They contain antioxidants that are essential for cognitive function. Low in fructose, berries are one of the most nutritious fruit options for young ones. Make sure berries are chopped or mashed, as whole berries can pose a choking risk.

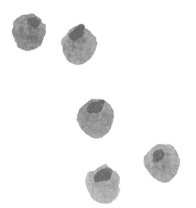

12 WHOLEGRAINS

A diet rich in wholegrains has been shown to reduce the risk of heart disease, type 2 diabetes, obesity and even cancer in later life. Wholegrains also improve digestive health by promoting the growth of beneficial bacteria in the colon. When we eat wholegrains, we digest plant-based protein, fibre, vitamins, minerals and a variety of phytochemicals that help improve our health. Stock your pantry with wholemeal staples such as brown rice, quinoa and wholemeal flour.

13 AVOCADO

Loaded with fibre, avocados also contain lots of 'good' fats. They are extremely versatile and make a nutritious and tasty addition to breakfast, lunch and dinner (see Holy Guacamole page 161).

14 LINSEED (FLAXSEED)

Good for brain and body, linseed contains ALA, selenium and fibre. ALA helps boost the brain's processing speed. The combination of selenium and fibre helps keep the digestive system on track, ensuring a happy bowel and a happy baby. Make sure linseeds are ground down, as whole or chopped linseeds pose a choking risk. Ground linseed is a great addition to most purées and is especially delicious stirred into your baby's morning porridge. Most supermarkets sell ground linseed in the health-food aisle.

15 GARLIC

Garlic contains antioxidants that support the body's protective mechanisms against oxidative damage. Garlic can significantly boost the function of the immune system, which is why you will notice that nearly all of the savoury recipes in this book include garlic.

16 OATS

Oats aid digestion and release energy slowly – perfect for keeping young tummies satisfied for longer. Porridge is always a good way to include oats in baby's diet.

17 QUINOA

Quinoa is one of the only plant-based foods that contains all nine essential amino acids that are the building blocks of muscle growth. Quinoa is also very high in antioxidants and contains almost twice as much fibre as other grains. Make sure you thoroughly rinse quinoa before cooking. See our great quinoa breakfast options to help get your baby started on the good stuff.

18 CHIA SEEDS

A great source of omega–3 fatty acids, chia seeds are loaded with nutrients that benefit body and brain. They can help regulate blood-sugar levels and are great for the intestinal tract, keeping your little one regular. Their mild flavour makes them the ideal versatile ingredient to add to food or drinks. Also add to yoghurt, purées, rice dishes, smoothies and baked goods. See our breakfast recipes (page 90) for ideas on how to build chia into your baby's diet.

19 DARK LEAFY GREENS

Rich in folate, iron, fibre and vitamins C and K, leafy greens are the immune system's ambrosia. If your young one tends to fall sick often, increase their intake of greens to naturally strengthen their immunity.

20 YOGHURT

Probiotics are essential for optimal gut health, which in turn stimulates the immune system. Greek-style yoghurt has less sugar and two to three times the amount of protein than regular yoghurt, so seek out this variety. It's so versatile: Greek yoghurt can be used as a marinade, sauce, dip, dessert and even in a drink.

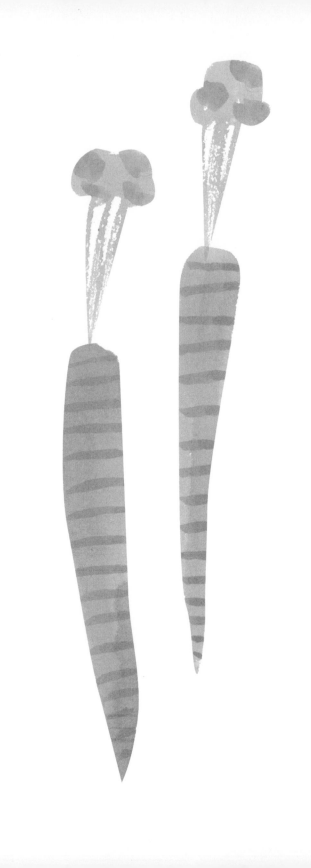

THE
NOT-SO-FUN
SIDE OF
SOLIDS

CHAPTER 3

FOOD REFUSAL

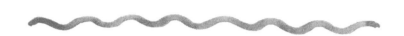

Babies are often cautious when introduced to new foods and this might lead them to reject some of the food you want to feed them. Of course, the food you'd rather they didn't eat (that interesting looking bug they just found in the grass, or that crust from breakfast you missed on the floor) are enormously tasty to them and will be wolfed down before you can blink an eye.

It's important to be patient and persistent when trying new food on babies. Be aware that some babies might just prefer to skip the mushy food stage altogether and go straight to finger foods when they are ready. There can also be valid reasons why your baby is having trouble accepting solid food.

Here are some of those reasons:

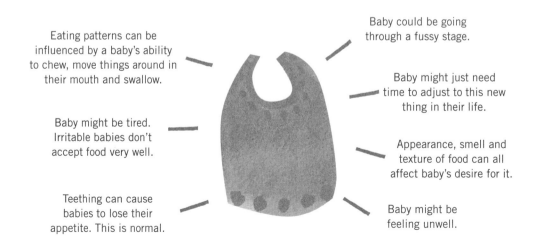

Eating patterns can be influenced by a baby's ability to chew, move things around in their mouth and swallow.

Baby might be tired. Irritable babies don't accept food very well.

Teething can cause babies to lose their appetite. This is normal.

Baby could be going through a fussy stage.

Baby might just need time to adjust to this new thing in their life.

Appearance, smell and texture of food can all affect baby's desire for it.

Baby might be feeling unwell.

OPTIONS FOR HANDLING FOOD REFUSAL

OPTION 1

Hide in your closet and curl up in the foetal position. Actually, we don't seriously recommend this. We much prefer Option 2.

OPTION 2

- Be persistent and calm. It might take several attempts before baby will accept the new food.

- Avoid introducing new foods when your child is tired or irritable.

- Try offering half a milk feed and then half a solid feed.

- Try offering or mixing the new flavour with an established favourite.

- Pay attention to how your baby enjoys their food: some like to play with their food and some prefer to feed themselves, especially around the nine-month mark.

- Let baby see you smiling while you are eating the same food.

- Ensure the food is not too hot. Lukewarm or room temperature is best.

If after the age of seven to nine months your infant still doesn't want to accept solids, it might be a good idea to consult your doctor who can refer you to a specialist, including a paediatrician or speech pathologist if needed. When in doubt, always seek the advice of a qualified health professional. The information in this, or any other, book should not replace the advice given by your doctor.

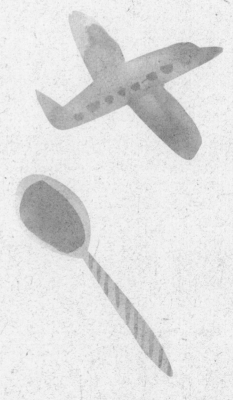

CONSTIPATION & CURES

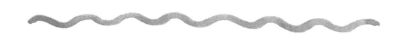

Remember the days when you considered bowel movements to be inappropriate dinner conversation or icebreakers when you met new people? Well, things have changed now you're a parent. There will be days when this is the only conversational topic you have to offer. You know you've reached this new level of intimacy when you talk to total strangers about the size, texture, smell and consistency of your little darling's poo.

"Oh, what a lovely baby," coos the sweet old lady who steps into the lift with you. "You must be very proud. Is she sleeping and eating well?"

"Oh, yes," you reply. "She sleeps well, eats well. Wonderful bowel movements. Such a lovely texture. Smooth yet solid. Fine-grained rather than coarse. And the colour – oh, the colour – a light latte with bold strokes of walnut, interspersed with flecks of russet and finished with an auburn twist."

You gaze fondly into the pram, unaware that your new friend is edging away from you, eyes fixed desperately on the lift doors.

And then you reach a new milestone. Constipation. If you thought you had lost every shred of self-respect with your bowel-movement conversation, wait until the day your baby gets constipation and you suddenly stop in a crowd, unconsciously mimicking the contortions of the blocked-up infant face. Ah yes, we'll stop at nothing to encourage our little ones to expel that pellet-like bowel motion, especially if they have been constipated for a while.

Don't despair. Most parents have been there and done that. It's actually quite common for babies to suffer constipation during the transition from milk to solids. Sometimes babies can go for days without a bowel movement. This is normal as long as their stools are wet rather than dry and hard.

SIGNS OF CONSTIPATION

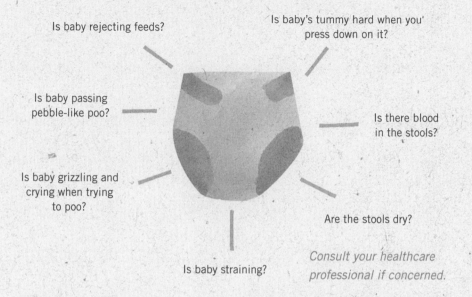

Is baby rejecting feeds?

Is baby's tummy hard when you' press down on it?

Is baby passing pebble-like poo?

Is there blood in the stools?

Is baby grizzling and crying when trying to poo?

Are the stools dry?

Is baby straining?

Consult your healthcare professional if concerned.

FOODS THAT MIGHT CAUSE CONSTIPATION

- Unripe bananas
- Rice cereal
- Cheese
- Potato
- White flour or bread
- Pasta

CURES FOR CONSTIPATION

- Add fibrous foods into baby's diet.
- Encourage baby to drink 30 ml (1 fl oz) cooled boiled water between feeds.
- Give baby a warm bath and gentle tummy massage.
- Lay baby on their back and gently rotate their legs in a circular motion.

FOODS THAT ARE DO-ABLE & POO-ABLE

These easy-to-digest foods might help move things along:

- Peaches
- Pears
- Prunes
- Avocado
- Plums
- Sweet potato
- Ground flaxseeds
- Spinach
- Beans
- Yoghurt

CHOKING & FIRST AID

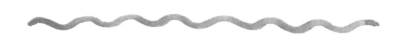

Many babies gag as they go through the mechanics of swallowing food rather than liquid. The first time it happens you might find yourself ripping baby from the high chair, turning them upside down, shoving your fingers down their throat and whacking them frantically on the back while your partner ricochets across the room, dials emergency and screams hysterically into the phone. And all of this in 2.5 seconds.

This is a normal reaction for first-time parents but not such a great thing for bub, who is now shrieking and has developed a morbid fear of mashed potato. There is a big difference between gagging and choking, and learning to recognise the difference can make mealtimes less like an episode of *Grey's Anatomy*.

Gagging is usually a temporary situation and should resolve itself naturally and quickly. We tend to recognise it as being messy and noisy while choking is normally (but not always) silent. Choking occurs when the airway becomes blocked and prevents breathing. When someone is choking they might start to cough and then become silent and unable to cough, cry or speak.

We highly recommend attending a Child Safety and First Aid Course to be fully trained in the correct response to choking and other emergencies. Make sure to place the first-aid kit where you have easy access to it in an emergency.

AVOIDING CHOKING HAZARDS

- Always supervise your baby when they are eating or drinking.

- Ensure baby is in an upright position when eating.

- Cut food into small pieces, especially the most common choking foods, such as grapes.

- Delay introducing foods that are difficult to swallow while your child is still small and learning the mechanics of swallowing solid food.

- Never force food into a child's mouth.

Start with silky-smooth soft purées at around six months of age and progress to lumpy and mushy textures, then onto finger foods as your child's eating skills develop. See the Developmental Eating Guide on page 38.

DENTAL HYGIENE

Having teeth brushed can be quite disconcerting for a baby, so it makes sense to get your infant used to dental hygiene from an early age. Before your baby even has teeth, start getting them used to the sensation by running a soft clean flannel or face cloth gently over their gums. When your baby's teeth start to emerge, brush gently twice a day with a soft toothbrush.

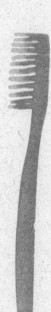

TIPS FOR TEETH BRUSHING

- Let baby watch you brushing your own teeth with your toothbrush, then try putting their toothbrush in their mouth. Chances are they will be curious enough to try it and seeing you doing it first will reduce the element of surprise or fear.

- If baby is not opening their mouth for you, let them see you with your mouth wide open. Before you know it, they will have copied you and opened their mouth too. A great tip for the sleep-deprived and yawning parent!

- Be very gentle.

- Sit baby in front of you and get their attention. When they tilt their head back to look at you, insert the toothbrush. This position enables you to see and gain access to all of the teeth.

THE DEVELOPMENTAL EATING GUIDE

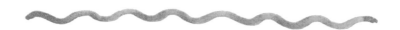

Babies will all vary in the time they need to progress through each stage of the developmental eating guide. By offering a wide variety of tastes and textures appropriate to their stage of development, you will help develop both their taste preferences and their oral motor skills.

SMOOTH STAGE

- Around six months of age
- Smooth purées that have a thin smooth texture, similar to the consistency of runny custard

LUMPY STAGE

- Around seven months of age
- Lumpy mashes, thicker purées and mashed meals
- Baby might be showing readiness to start on finger foods

FINGER FOOD STAGE

- Around eight months of age or when baby is able to sit upright with little or no support and grasp objects

- Encourage your baby to feed themselves by offering a variety of soft finger foods

- Cut food into small pieces that can easily be managed or held onto while baby is chewing

- Avoid potential choking risks such as raw carrot, celery, apple, or small whole foods such as grapes, nuts and pieces of sausage. However, these can all be offered if chopped or mashed.

- At the start, baby might treat finger food more as a plaything than a food. As the weeks progress, however, you will find the food moves from being chomped on and played with to finally being swallowed.

- Starter finger food options include soft cooked fruit and vegetable fingers, frittata fingers, grated cheese, soft fingers of banana or avocado, and flaky fish bites.

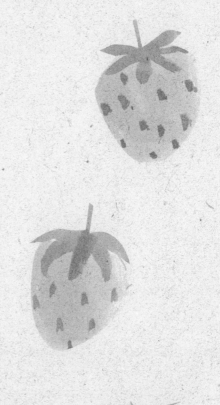

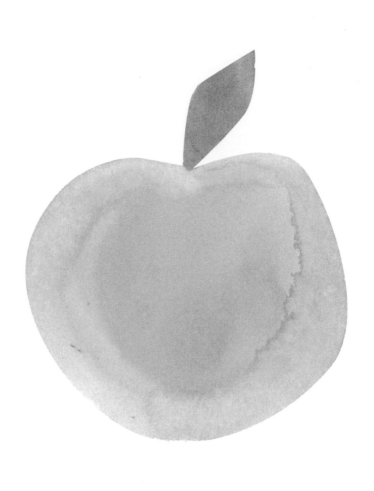

Staples to keep you sane

Chapter 4

TO COOK WITH

- Steaming basket
- Small to medium saucepans with lids
- Frying pan
- Baking paper
- Handheld blender
- Food processor
- Measuring cups and spoons
- Scales
- Quality vegetable peeler (you will be peeling a lot!)
- Grater
- Whisk

TO STORE WITH

- Ice-cube trays with lids
- Resealable freezer bags
- Airtight containers (look for BPA-free)
- Marker pen

TO EAT WITH

- Highchair with infant support cushion
- Bibs (dishwasher-safe plastic bibs and ones with a catching lip are great for saving clean-up time)
- Plastic bowls (you will need a billion of these – hello IKEA!)
- Spoons (always use silicone or plastic spoons as metal spoons can burn baby's mouth)
- Face cloths and flannels (towelling cloths are gentler on baby's new skin than commercial baby wipes)

STOCKING UP

IN YOUR FREEZER

Have spinach, broccoli, corn, peas, blueberries, raspberries.

Frozen fruit and vegetables are easy to prepare – just wash, chop, throw in a resealable plastic bag and freeze. Wherever possible, use organically grown fruit and vegetables.

IN YOUR FRIDGE

Have meat, fish, poultry, cheese, yoghurt, eggs, fruit and vegetables (lots of the good green stuff) and fresh herbs.

IN YOUR PANTRY

Have tinned beans (try to make sure the lining of the tin is BPA-free), wholewheat pasta, brown rice, quinoa, oats, salt-reduced broth (gluten-free if you prefer; you can make your own and store in the freezer), nuts, wholemeal couscous, wholemeal flour, chia seeds, LSA, tinned salmon and tuna, rice noodles, coconut oil, coconut milk and cream, lentils, dried herbs and ground spices (cumin, coriander, cinnamon, ginger, nutmeg, oregano, Italian mixed herbs, rosemary, thyme and tarragon).

HOW TO COOK

STEAMING

Steaming is the best way to retain nutrients, so steam food as often as possible. If you don't have a steaming basket, use a metal colander over a saucepan of boiling water.

BOILING

Boiling is a very simple way of cooking, but be mindful of overcooking as it can destroy important nutrients. Minimise the loss of nutrients by boiling in minimal water and re-using the cooking water when blending.

BLENDING

A small food processor or handheld blender is efficient to use, small to store and also very easy to clean.

REHEATING

Reheat thawed or refrigerated meals in a microwave oven or in a small amount of water in a saucepan. Ensure the food has been heated to at least 70°C (160°F). Stir the food during the reheating process to ensure even distribution of heat. Once reheated, test the temperature before giving it to your baby. Always throw away any leftover reheated food.

RECIPE INFORMATION AT A GLANCE

Each recipe has an easy-to-read key showing preparation and cooking times, serving quantities and suitability for freezing.

 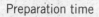
Preparation time

Cooking time

Serving quantity

Good to freeze

HOW TO STORE

FRIDGE

Cover, cool and refrigerate cooked food immediately. To hasten the cooling process, store in shallow containers. As soon as it is cooled, transfer to the freezer or refrigerator. If refrigerating, make sure containers are airtight and discard the contents if not used within two days.

FREEZER

When you have cooked a purée, add a little more boiled water and then immediately freeze in small portions, using an ice-cube tray. Once frozen, pop out the ice cubes and put them in a freezerproof resealable plastic bag. Label each bag with the ingredients and the date. Every evening take out the portion you plan to use the next day and put it in the fridge to defrost overnight. Do not refreeze meals that have already been thawed and, if in doubt, throw it out. It's not worth risking a bout of tummy troubles or worse.

RECOMMENDED FOOD STORAGE GUIDE

	FRIDGE	FREEZER
Meat	1 day	1 month
Meat & vegetable combination	1–2 days	1 month
Cooked fruits & vegetables	2–3 days	1 month

To be on the safe side we advise storing any baby food in the freezer for a maximum of 1 month.

CAULIFLOWER RICE

Forget white rice; cauli-rice is just as nice!

1 large cauliflower

1 Start by taking any leaves off the cauliflower, then cut the cauliflower into quarters. Cut out the central stem (this can be reserved to eat as a crunchy snack with a nice avocado dip).

2 Bring a large saucepan of salted water to the boil and add the cauliflower quarters. Simmer for 20 minutes, then strain and set aside to cool.

3 Using a coarse grater or food processor, either grate the cauliflower or pulse until it has a rice-like texture. You might end up with a couple of larger chunks but that is okay. Season with salt and pepper.

4 To reheat, put the cauliflower rice in a microwave bowl and cover with plastic wrap. Microwave on High for 2 minutes. (Add a little butter to the rice to keep it moist and give it a lovely flavour.)

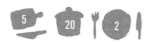

BAKED SWEET POTATO CHIPS

There's no need to feel guilty when eating these delicious chips that are packed with vitamins.

2 unpeeled sweet potatoes (kumara), scrubbed
2 tablespoons olive oil
Sprig of fresh thyme, leaves picked
1 teaspoon garlic powder

1 Cut each sweet potato in half lengthways, then in half again so each one becomes 8 large wedges.

2 Preheat the oven to 200°C (400°F). Line a baking tray with baking paper.

3 Whisk together the oil, thyme leaves and garlic powder and brush the chips on all sides. Spread the chips over the tray and bake for 45 minutes or until golden brown.

4 Season with salt and pepper.

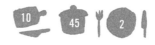

CHILD-FRIENDLY CONFIT GARLIC

Add confit garlic to any dish; there's no need to fry it. This is great, not only for kids, but also for people who don't like a strong garlic flavour.

500 g (1 lb 2 oz) garlic cloves, peeled
500 ml (17 fl oz/2 cups) olive oil

1 Preheat the oven to 160°C (315°F).

2 Put the garlic cloves in a deep baking dish and cover with olive oil so the garlic is completely submerged (add more oil if needed).

3 Cover the dish with foil and bake for 2½ hours until golden.

4 Strain the garlic, keeping the oil for other cooking.

5 Transfer the garlic to a food processor and blend to a smooth paste. Add a few tablespoons of the oil for a smoother consistency if needed.

6 Store in an airtight container in the fridge for up to 5 weeks.

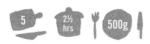

ZOODLE PASTA

Don't know what to feed the teeny-weenies? Just whip up this fantastic zucchini linguine.

2 zucchini (courgettes)
2 teaspoons olive oil
Shaved parmesan cheese (optional)

1 Trim the ends off the zucchini. Using a grater on a flat surface, slide the zucchini along the grater to form the noodles. When you get to the seeds, turn to the next side, until all four sides have been grated.

2 Heat the oil in a saucepan over medium heat and lightly fry the noodles for 1 minute. Add 3 tablespoons water and cook over low heat for a further 5–7 minutes. Season and serve hot with shaved parmesan, if using.

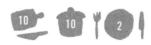

Veg It Up

It's easy to get stuck in a rut and keep serving the same vegetables every night, especially if you know your child will eat them; however, if you want to maximise your child's health now and in the future, mix it up a bit and offer them a rainbow of vegetables instead. Vegetables come in all colours, shapes and sizes, so dish up the full spectrum once they start eating solid food. Not only will the variety of colours appeal to them, but you will be boosting nutrition, developing their taste preferences and helping to prevent future fussiness.

These versatile vegetable dishes can be offered as a stand-alone meal or paired with your protein of choice. They are perfect for baby's lunchtime meals or as colourful accompaniments to main meals.

SUPERCHARGED MASH

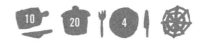

Who doesn't love mash? It's usually a favourite with kids, so we've supercharged the traditional mash: you can be sure that every bite is packed with nutrients.

210 g (7½ oz/1½ cups) sweet potato, peeled and chopped
3 carrots, peeled and chopped
3 parsnips, peeled and chopped
2 turnips, peeled and chopped
75 g (2¾ oz/1½ cups) spinach leaves
3 tablespoons milk
1 tablespoon butter
2 tablespoons finely chopped flat-leaf (Italian) parsley leaves

1 Combine all of the root vegetables in a large saucepan of water and boil for about 20 minutes until soft and cooked through.

2 Add the spinach and boil for 1 minute. Strain and discard the water.

3 Mash the vegetables with the milk and butter.

4 Stir in the parsley just before serving.

FOR BABY:

Purée to desired consistency. Don't forget to regularly offer different combinations of vegetables to help develop those tiny taste buds.

ALL GROWN UP:

Season with salt and pepper and serve with your favourite protein.

SMART TIP
Turnips are high in vitamin C and can help stimulate the immune system.

ROAST VEGETABLE CHIPS

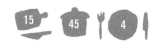

Kids love chips, don't they? But whoever thought they could be a nutritious choice? We've 'smartened up' the humble potato chip, so there's no need to feel guilty when you put a plate of these in front of the kids: it's a great way to get them to eat a variety of vegetables. Serve these up and watch them disappear!

4 tablespoons olive oil
1 handful pine nuts, crushed
1½ teaspoons fresh thyme leaves
50 g (1½ oz/½ cup) finely grated parmesan cheese
1 small beetroot (beet), peeled and cut into batons
1 carrot, peeled and cut into batons
1 small sweet potato, peeled and cut into batons
1 small zucchini (courgette), cut into batons
1 small parsnip, peeled and cut into batons

1 Preheat the oven to 180°C (350°F). Line a baking tray with baking paper.

2 Meanwhile, combine the olive oil, pine nuts, thyme and parmesan in a bowl. Stir to combine.

3 Spread the vegetable batons over the baking tray. Brush the pine nut mixture all over the batons. Bake for 45 minutes or until golden brown.

FOR BABY:

Children love to dip, so pair these chips with a lovely avocado dip (see page 161).

ALL GROWN UP:

Season with salt and pepper. Great for a snack or as a side dish.

SMART TIP

Beetroot is high in immune-boosting vitamins and is thought to improve oxygenation to the brain.

MINTY MUSHY PEAS

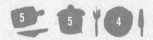

Believe it or not, comfort food is not always bad for you! This side dish is a delicious accompaniment to fish or a roast dinner. It's pure mushy comfort all the way, and the best thing about it is you can serve it to baby and the rest of the family without making any changes.

4 tablespoons unsalted
  butter
2 sprigs of mint, leaves
  picked
560 g (1 lb 4 oz/4 cups)
  frozen peas
½ lemon
2 tablespoons sour cream,
  or to taste

1 Melt the butter in a saucepan over low heat.
   Add the mint and peas, then cover and simmer
   for 5 minutes.

2 Add a squeeze of lemon juice, then mash the peas
   by hand or in a food processor.

3 Stir in the sour cream.

FOR BABY:

Serve with grilled fish.

ALL GROWN UP:

Season with salt and pepper and serve with grilled fish.

SMART TIP

With anti-inflammatory properties, peas are pint-sized powerhouses of nutrition. Try saying that three times fast!

CAULI-RICE SALAD

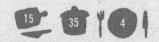

Can't get your mini-me to eat salad? Don't stress. Offer them this and they'll be begging for more!

1 cauliflower
155 g (5½ oz/1 cup) chopped pumpkin (squash)
140 g (5 oz/1 cup) chopped sweet potato
4 tablespoons coconut oil, melted
3 tablespoons sultanas, chopped to avoid choking risk
65 g (2½ oz/½ cup) crumbled feta cheese
80 g (2¾ oz/½ cup) pine nuts, crushed
2 tablespoons chopped flat-leaf (Italian) parsley

1 Preheat the oven to 180°C (350°F). Line a baking tray with baking paper.

2 Chop the cauliflower and process in a food processor to a rice-like texture.

3 Spread the pumpkin and sweet potato over the tray and drizzle with the coconut oil. Roast for 30 minutes or until soft and slightly golden.

4 Remove from the oven and mix in the cauliflower rice and sultanas. Return to the oven and cook for a further 5 minutes.

5 Stir in the feta, pine nuts and parsley to serve.

FOR BABY:

Purée to desired consistency or serve as a finger food.

ALL GROWN UP:

Season with salt and pepper and drizzle with a little honey for extra flavour.

SMART TIP
Cauliflower is an important source of vitamin C and choline. Choline can help boost brain function and improve learning and memory.

ROASTED RATATOUILLE

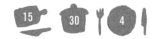

Roasting brings out the sweetness in the vegetables that make up this delicious side dish. The true beauty of it lies in its versatility, so try some of the serving suggestions below.

1 small eggplant (aubergine), cut into bite-size pieces

1 small zucchini (courgette), cut into bite-size pieces

1 red onion, coarsely chopped

1 yellow capsicum (pepper), cut into bite-size pieces

2 tablespoons olive oil

2 garlic cloves, crushed

2 tablespoons coarsely chopped flat-leaf (Italian) parsley

2 large roma tomatoes, coarsely chopped

2 teaspoons lemon juice

1 Preheat the oven to 200°C (400°F). Lightly grease a baking dish and put in the eggplant, zucchini, onion and capsicum.

2 In a small bowl, combine the olive oil, garlic and parsley. Drizzle over the vegetables and roast for 20 minutes or until the vegetables are tender.

3 When the vegetables are a light golden brown, mix in the tomato and lemon juice. Return to the oven and roast for a further 10 minutes or until the tomato is juicy.

FOR BABY:

Purée with a serving of polenta for a plant-based meal.

ALL GROWN UP:

Season with salt and pepper, then pair it with a protein, stir it through pasta or serve it on top of polenta or a piece of ciabatta with some crumbled feta cheese. Makes a fabulous side dish for breakfast, lunch or dinner.

SMART TIP

Tomatoes are packed with beneficial phytochemicals that play an important role in helping to prevent chronic disease.

GREEN VEGETABLE GRATIN

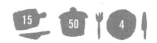

Start baby off on the good green stuff and you will not have a revolt on your hands when toddlerhood hits.

1 leek, finely chopped
1 zucchini (courgette), finely chopped
½ red cabbage, finely chopped
1 cup Super Power Pesto (page 135) or ready-made basil pesto
2 tablespoons olive oil
2 tablespoons finely grated parmesan cheese
1 slice wholemeal bread
1 handful pine nuts, crushed

1 Preheat the oven to 180°C (350°F). Line a baking tray with baking paper.

2 Put the leek, zucchini and cabbage in a large bowl. Stir in the pesto with 1 tablespoon of the olive oil, making sure all ingredients are well coated.

3 Spread over the tray and bake for 20 minutes.

4 Meanwhile, make the topping by processing the parmesan and bread in a food processor until it has a nice crumbly texture – not too fine.

5 Scatter the cheese mixture and pine nuts over the vegetable mixture and bake for a further 10 minutes or until golden on top.

FOR BABY:

Purée to the desired consistency. Mix in some protein for a well-rounded meal.

ALL GROWN UP:

Season with salt and pepper and pair with lamb chops.

SMART TIP

Red cabbage is high in antioxidants and anthocyanins that can improve brain function.

RESCUE REMEDIES

Many traditional foods can provide health benefits. We have put together a list of common baby concerns and suggested some remedy purées to help you in caring for your child.

A GOOD NIGHT'S SLEEP

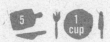

The elusive sleep fairy has vanished once again. Don't despair: create your own magic with this recipe and help send bub off to dreamland.

1 banana
½ avocado
155 g (5½ oz/1 cup) blueberries
1 tablespoon Greek-style yoghurt
1 teaspoon LSA meal (linseed, sunflower seed and almond meal)

1 Use a food processor or handheld blender to purée all the ingredients with a little breastmilk or formula.

2 Store in an airtight container in the fridge for 1 day.

SMART TIP
Bananas, yoghurt and nuts all contain high levels of tryptophan, which has a sedative effect, promoting sleepiness and relaxation. Feed your baby this purée just before bedtime.

CONSTIPATION CURE

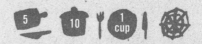

If bub has a case of 'too much strain with no gain' then it's time to ease things along a little with this recipe.

55 g (2 oz/¼ cup) pitted prunes

80 g (2¾ oz/½ cup) tinned chickpeas (garbanzo beans), rinsed

2 tablespoons plain yoghurt

1 Steam the prunes in a steaming basket until plumped up and very tender. Transfer to a food processor or handheld blender to purée with the chickpeas.

2 Add the yoghurt and blend well, unless you want to freeze the mixture. If freezing, thaw and add a small amount of yoghurt to each portion.

3 Freeze in individual portions for up to 1 month or store in an airtight container in the fridge for 1 day.

SMART TIP

Chickpeas are praised for their high fibre content and prunes have a mild laxative effect, both of which can help bub stay regular and relieve constipation.

TEETHING RELIEF

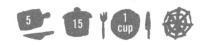

If the Teething Fairy (the Tooth Fairy's evil twin) is visiting, whip up this dish.

60 g (2¼ oz/½ cup)
  broccoli florets
1 pear, peeled, cored and
  coarsely chopped
½ teaspoon finely chopped
  fresh tarragon

1 Steam the broccoli florets in a steaming basket for 10 minutes. Add the pear to the basket and steam for 5 minutes or until all ingredients are tender.

2 Use a food processor or handheld blender to purée with the tarragon and a little bit of cooking liquid to reach the desired consistency.

3 Freeze in individual portions for up to 1 month or store in an airtight container in the fridge for 1 day.

SMART TIP

Tarragon helps soothe toothache and promotes a good night's sleep – a winning combination for all.

IMMUNITY BOOSTER

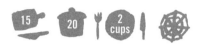

Pep up the whole family's immune system and keep the bad bugs at bay with this recipe.

1 carrot, peeled and
  chopped
½ sweet potato, peeled and
  chopped
1 beetroot (beet), peeled
  and chopped
2 teaspoons olive oil
½ teaspoon fresh thyme
  leaves

1 Preheat the oven to 180°C (350°F). Line a baking tray with baking paper.

2 Spread the vegetables over the tray, drizzle with the olive oil and sprinkle with thyme leaves. Roast for 20 minutes or until cooked through and tender.

3 Transfer to a food processor or use a handheld blender to purée to the desired consistency.

4 Freeze in individual portions for up to 1 month or store in an airtight container in the fridge for 1 day.

SMART TIP

Root vegetables are packed with phytonutrients and fibre, essential for overall health.

HAPPY TUMMY

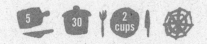

Happy tummies equal happy mummies so get bub's digestive juices going. This recipe pairs well with any protein.

½ sweet potato, peeled and chopped
2 tablespoons olive oil
2 teaspoons butter
½ small onion, finely chopped
1 garlic clove, crushed
¼ teaspoon ground coriander
¼ teaspoon ground cumin
100 g (3½ oz/½ cup) red lentils, rinsed
375 ml (13 fl oz/1½ cups) salt-reduced vegetable stock
Greek-style yoghurt (optional)

1 Preheat the oven to 180°C (350°F). Line a baking tray with baking paper.

2 Spread the sweet potato over the tray and drizzle with olive oil. Bake for 30 minutes or until tender.

3 Meanwhile, melt the butter in a small saucepan over medium heat. Add the onion and sauté for 5 minutes. Add the garlic and cook for 1 minute. Now add the spices and stir for 30 seconds. Stir in the lentils and add the stock. Simmer, covered, for 20 minutes, stirring occasionally.

4 When the stock has been absorbed and the lentils are mushy, remove from the heat and stir in the sweet potato.

5 Cool a little and add a dollop of yoghurt, if using.

6 Freeze in individual portions for up to 1 month (without the yoghurt) or store in an airtight container in the fridge for 1 day.

SMART TIP
Lentils are a high-protein food and are fantastic for digestive health.

STRONG BONES

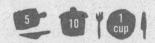

New little bones will get a good supply of calcium (for health and strength) with this purée.

100 g (3½ oz/2 cups) spinach leaves, destemmed

100 g (3½ oz/½ cup) tinned sweet corn kernels, rinsed

115 g (4 oz/½ cup) ricotta cheese

¼ teaspoon freshly grated nutmeg

1 Steam the spinach leaves in a steaming basket until slightly wilted. Allow to cool.

2 Put the spinach, corn, ricotta and nutmeg in a food processor or use a handheld blender to purée to the desired consistency.

3 Not suitable to freeze. Store in an airtight container in the fridge for up to 1 day.

SMART TIP

Ricotta is a good choice for a calcium hit as it is low in sodium and high in vitamins A and B and zinc.

BRAIN POWER

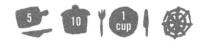

This little brain booster is tasty, nutritious and easy to make.

2 green apples, peeled, cored and chopped

25 g (1 oz/½ cup) spinach, destemmed

75 g (2¾ oz/½ cup) frozen peas

½ teaspoon finely chopped fresh mint

1 Steam the apples, spinach and peas in a steaming basket for 10 minutes or until tender.

2 Transfer to a food processor or use a handheld blender to purée with the mint. Add a little bit of cooking liquid, if needed.

3 Freeze in individual portions for up to 1 month or store in an airtight container in the fridge for 1 day.

SMART TIP

Spinach is a rich source of non-haem iron. At around six months of age, baby's natural iron reserves start to diminish, making it crucial that they receive adequate amounts of iron-rich foods to help support healthy brain development.

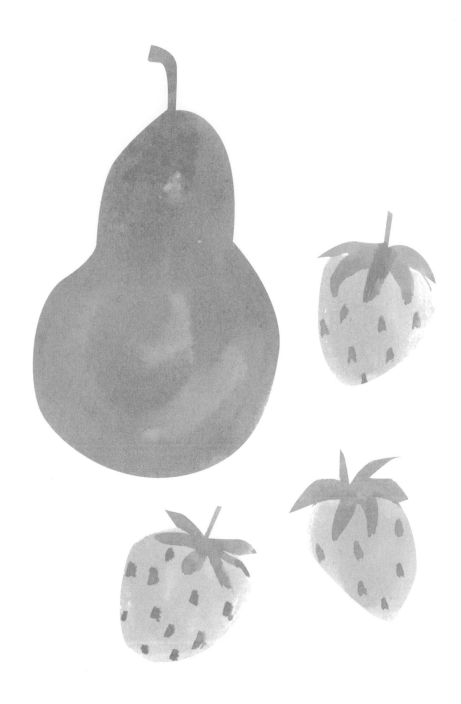

FIRST
TASTES

CHAPTER 5

HOW TO START

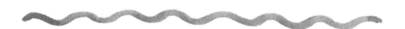

You are now ready to begin introducing your baby to solid food, using the purées featured in this chapter. To make the process easier for both of you, we have included these top 10 tips:

1   Choose a time during the day (usually around lunchtime) when your mini-me is feeling rested and happy. Another reason for choosing the middle of the day is that, if an allergic reaction occurs, it will be easier to monitor during daylight hours.

2   You might like to offer some breastmilk or formula first. Try half a normal feed. It takes the edge off their hunger and prevents them feeling frustrated. A frustrated baby is more likely to refuse food.

3   Start with 1–2 teaspoons of lukewarm, silky-smooth purée (refer to our First Tastes Meal Plan on page 67). Always test the temperature before offering it to baby and don't use a metal spoon, which can retain heat and also feel hard and sharp in an infant's mouth.

4   Put a little purée on a silicone spoon and gently place it in baby's mouth. Baby should allow you to spoonfeed them; later on, they will grab the spoon and try to feed themselves.

5   If bub shuts their mouth and turns their head, do not force them to eat. It's important to remain patient and happy. You want to show that this is an enjoyable part of life. If it's really not working, you might need to stop and try again tomorrow.

6   Putting some purée on the tip of your finger might encourage your mini-me to suck the purée off your finger.

7   Playing with food is an important learning experience so get the face cloths ready (and the camera).

8   Progress slowly, building up from 1 teaspoon and following
    the amounts on page 66. Tiny tummies need time to adjust
    and metabolise this new food. You can always top it up with
    breastmilk or formula if baby is still hungry.

9   It is essential that baby begins to receive iron-rich foods by
    the time they are six months old. If they don't, there could be
    implications for their neurocognitive development. Rice cereal
    is typically the first food offered to babies, as it is fortified with
    iron. If you want to skip the rice cereal, make sure you include
    a lot of iron-rich foods, such as puréed meat, poultry, cooked
    plain tofu, legumes and beans.

10 Use our Meal Planners to guide you through the first few
    months of starting solids. Our recipes are optimised for health
    and nutrition. They begin with simple purées with a focus
    on introducing protein, vegetables, fruit, grains, legumes
    and 'good' fats for best digestion and nutrient uptake. Once
    foods have been gradually introduced and any potential food
    intolerances have been identified, children can and should eat
    the same foods as adults with slight adjustments to exclude
    salt and foods listed as unsafe (see our Food & Drinks to Avoid
    section on page 17).

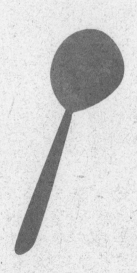

FIRST TASTES MEAL PLAN

This chapter is full of ideas for starter purées that can be served as first solid foods. Every baby is different, so use the quantities suggested as a guide only. On the first day, start with just 1 TEASPOON of purée around lunchtime that day.

Every day increase the amount consumed by 1 teaspoon until, around the four- or five-day mark, baby is consuming roughly 1 TABLESPOON a day.

Once baby has mastered that, introduce a second daily meal of 1 teaspoon. Gradually increase to 2–4 tablespoons per meal and progress to 3 meals per day. This process could take 1–2 months.

Continue breastfeeding or giving formula during this time. In the chart opposite we have called this a 'milk feed'.

FIRST TASTES MEAL PLAN

	EARLY MORNING	MID MORNING	LUNCH	EVENING	BEDTIME
DAY 1	Milk feed	Milk feed	Milk feed followed by carrot purée	Milk feed	Milk feed
DAY 2	Milk feed	Milk feed	Milk feed followed by avocado purée	Milk feed	Milk feed
DAY 3	Milk feed	Milk feed	Milk feed followed by carrot and avocado purée	Milk feed	Milk feed
DAY 4	Milk feed	Milk feed	Milk feed followed by sweet potato purée	Milk feed	Milk feed
DAY 5	Milk feed	Milk feed	Milk feed followed by sweet potato and broccoli purée	Milk feed	Milk feed
DAY 6	Milk feed	Milk feed	Milk feed followed by sweet potato and chicken purée	Milk feed	Milk feed
DAY 7	Milk feed	Milk feed	Milk feed followed by banana purée	Milk feed	Milk feed

STARTER FOODS

Did you know that babies have around 10,000 taste buds? That's twice as many as adults. The more we stimulate those taste buds by introducing new flavours, the more neural pathways are created. How wonderful that we can use this developmental stage to broaden baby's taste preference and boost brain function at the same time.

Consider the first few months as palate training. Start your baby off with one of the following starter purées for the first few tastes, but don't hesitate to progress to combining them soon after, with the aim of exposing your baby to as many flavours as possible. See the Pair It Up suggestions (pages 81–5) for some great combination ideas.

To give purées extra smart power, add a pinch of brain-boosting ground chia seeds, LSA meal or nut meal.

To help your infant develop good chewing skills, it's important to introduce them to texture gradually. When starting solids, make sure the texture is very smooth. Create a consistency somewhere between semi-liquid and runny custard. To thin a purée add a little cooled boiled water, breastmilk or formula.

Here are a few pointers:

- As your baby progresses, start to make purées lumpier and to introduce mashes. Stir in textural foods such as yoghurt, grated cheese, nut meal, well-cooked rice, quinoa, chia seeds and pasta. This is an important process in learning how to chew properly.

- If your child is having difficulty adjusting to solid food you might find they will accept lumpier purées or soft finger foods more readily than thinner purées.

- Offer variety by freezing single food purées and then mixing and matching them each day. Adding spices and herbs will also help broaden your baby's palate.

Vegetable Purées

BROCCOLI

250 g (9 oz) broccoli, chopped

1 Steam the broccoli in a steaming basket until florets are tender.

2 Use a food processor or handheld blender to purée with a little of the cooking liquid if needed to reach the desired consistency.

3 Freeze in individual portions for up to 1 month or store in an airtight container in the fridge for 1 day.

SPICE IT UP:

Purée with ¼ teaspoon snipped chives.

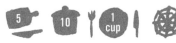

CARROT

2 carrots, peeled and coarsely chopped

1 Steam the carrot in a steaming basket until tender.

2 Use a food processor or handheld blender to purée with a little of the cooking liquid if needed to reach the desired consistency.

3 Freeze in individual portions for up to 1 month or store in an airtight container in the fridge for 1 day.

SPICE IT UP:

Add ¼ teaspoon ground ginger.

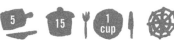

CAULIFLOWER

250 g (9 oz) cauliflower, cut into florets

1 Steam the cauliflower florets in a steaming basket until tender.

2 Use a food processor or handheld blender to purée with a little of the cooking liquid if needed to reach the desired consistency.

3 Freeze in individual portions for up to 1 month or store in an airtight container in the fridge for 1 day.

SPICE IT UP:

Add ¼ teaspoon of ground turmeric to the purée.

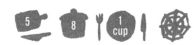

PARSNIP

1 parsnip, peeled and chopped
1 thyme sprig, leaves picked
Olive oil, for drizzling

1 Preheat the oven to 180°C (350°F). Line a baking tray with baking paper.

2 Toss the parsnip with thyme and olive oil to lightly coat and roast until caramelised and tender.

3 Use a food processor or handheld blender to purée, adding a little cooled boiled water if needed.

4 Freeze in individual portions for up to 1 month or store in an airtight container in the fridge for 1 day.

SPICE IT UP:

Add ½ teaspoon of finely chopped fresh thyme to the purée.

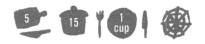

PEAS

250 g (9 oz) frozen peas

1 Put the peas in a saucepan with 2 tablespoons of water. Cover and cook over low heat for 6–8 minutes until tender.

2 Use a food processor or handheld blender to purée with a little of the cooking liquid if needed to reach the desired consistency.

3 Freeze in individual portions for up to 1 month or store in an airtight container in the fridge for 1 day.

SPICE IT UP:

Add ½ teaspoon of finely chopped fresh mint to the purée.

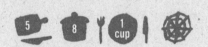

POTATO

2 purple-skinned potatoes, peeled and coarsely chopped

1 Steam the potato in a steaming basket until tender.

2 Use a food processor or handheld blender to purée with a little of the cooking liquid if needed to reach the desired consistency.

3 Freeze in individual portions for up to 1 month or store in an airtight container in the fridge for 1 day.

SPICE IT UP:

Add ½ teaspoon of finely chopped fresh tarragon to the purée.

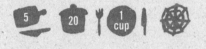

PUMPKIN

½ butternut pumpkin (squash), peeled, deseeded and chopped

1   Put the pumpkin in a saucepan with 2 tablespoons of water. Cover and cook over low heat for 6–8 minutes until tender. Alternatively, sprinkle the pumpkin with a little grated nutmeg and olive oil and roast in the oven at 180°C (350°F) until caramelised and cooked through.

2   Use a food processor or handheld blender to purée with a little of the cooking liquid to reach the desired consistency.

3   Freeze in individual portions for up to 1 month or store in an airtight container in the fridge for 1 day.

SPICE IT UP:

Add ¼ teaspoon of finely grated nutmeg to the purée.

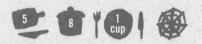

SPINACH

250 g (9 oz) spinach leaves, destemmed and coarsely chopped

1   Steam the spinach in a steaming basket until tender.

2   Use a food processor or handheld blender to purée with a little of the cooking liquid to reach the desired consistency.

3   Freeze in individual portions for up to 1 month or store in an airtight container in the fridge for 1 day.

SPICE IT UP:

Add ¼ teaspoon of finely chopped fresh dill to the purée.

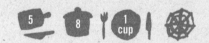

SWEET POTATO

1 sweet potato, peeled and coarsely chopped.

1 Steam the sweet potato in a steaming basket until tender.

2 Use a food processor or handheld blender to purée with a little of the cooking liquid to reach the desired consistency.

3 Freeze in individual portions for up to 1 month or store in an airtight container in the fridge for 1 day.

SPICE IT UP:

Add ¼ teaspoon of finely grated nutmeg to the purée.

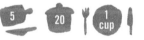

ZUCCHINI

1 zucchini (courgette), peeled and coarsely chopped

1 Steam the zucchini in a steaming basket until tender.

2 Use a food processor or handheld blender to purée with a little of the cooking liquid, if needed, to reach the desired consistency.

3 Freeze in individual portions for up to 1 month or store in an airtight container in the fridge for 1 day.

SPICE IT UP:

Add ½ teaspoon finely chopped fresh mint to the purée.

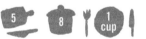

Fruit Purées

Apple

2 large apples, peeled, cored and chopped

1 Put the apple in a small saucepan with 2 tablespoons water. Cover and cook over low heat for 6–8 minutes until tender.

2 Use a food processor or handheld blender to purée with a little bit of the cooking liquid to reach the desired consistency.

3 Freeze in individual portions for up to 1 month or store in an airtight container in the fridge for 1 day.

SPICE IT UP:

Add ¼ teaspoon of ground cinnamon to the purée.

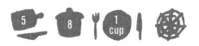

Apricot

425 g (15 oz) tin apricot halves in natural juice, drained
Greek-style yoghurt (optional)

1 Use a food processor or handheld blender to purée with a little yoghurt, if using.

2 Freeze in individual portions for up to 1 month (without yoghurt) or store in an airtight container in the fridge for 1 day.

SPICE IT UP:

Add ¼ teaspoon of ground cumin to the purée.

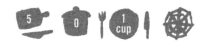

AVOCADO

1 avocado

1 Cut a wedge of avocado of the amount baby will eat, as once the stone is removed the avocado flesh will oxidise quickly and turn brown. Keep the remaining avocado.

2 Remove the skin from the wedge and mash the flesh with a fork, using a little breastmilk or formula to reach the desired consistency.

3 Store in the fridge for up to 1 day. Not suitable for freezing. Don't worry if the purée becomes a little discoloured after storing – it won't change the flavour.

SPICE IT UP:

Add ½ teaspoon of finely chopped fresh basil to the mash.

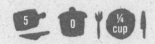

BANANA

2 bananas, peeled
Greek-style yoghurt

1 Process or blend the bananas until smooth. Alternatively, preheat the oven to 180°C (350°F). Line a baking tray with baking paper, cut the bananas in half lengthways and lay on the tray. Sprinkle with a little ground cinnamon and roast until slightly golden brown and caramelised. Cool down before mashing with a dollop of Greek-style yoghurt.

2 Freeze in individual portions (without yoghurt) for up to 1 month or store in an airtight container in the fridge for 1 day.

SPICE IT UP:

Add ¼ teaspoon of ground cinnamon to the purée.

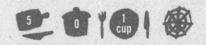

BLUEBERRY

155 g (5½ oz/1 cup) fresh blueberries
Greek-style yoghurt (optional)

1 Use a food processor or handheld
   blender to purée the berries with a
   little yoghurt, if using.

2 Freeze in individual portions (without
   yoghurt) for up to 1 month or store in
   the fridge for 1 day.

SPICE IT UP:

*Add ¼ teaspoon of ground cinnamon to
the purée.*

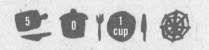

DATE

6 dates, pitted and coarsely chopped
Greek-style yoghurt (optional)

1 Steam the dates in a steaming basket
   until tender.

2 Transfer the dates to a food processor
   or use a handheld blender to purée
   with a little yoghurt, if using, to reach
   the desired consistency.

3 Freeze in individual portions for up to
   1 month (without yoghurt) or store in
   an airtight container in the fridge for
   1 day.

SPICE IT UP:

*Add ¼ teaspoon of ground cardamom to
the purée.*

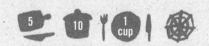

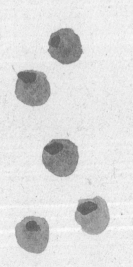

GRAPE

180 g (6¼ oz/1 cup) seedless grapes,
coarsely chopped

1 Use a food processor or handheld
blender to purée the grapes.

2 Freeze in individual portions for up
to 1 month or store in an airtight
container in the fridge for 1 day.

SPICE IT UP:

Add ½ teaspoon of fresh mint to
the purée.

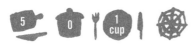

MANGO

2 mangoes

1 Coarsely chop the mango flesh and
use a food processor or handheld
blender to purée.

2 Freeze in individual portions for up
to 1 month or store in an airtight
container in the fridge for 1 day.

SPICE IT UP:

Add ½ teaspoon of finely chopped fresh
coriander (cilantro) to the purée.

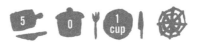

PEAR

2 large pears, peeled, cored and chopped

1 Steam the pears in a steaming basket until tender.

2 Use a food processor or handheld blender to purée with a little of the cooking liquid to reach the desired consistency.

3 Freeze in individual portions for up to 1 month or store in an airtight container in the fridge for 1 day.

SPICE IT UP:

Add ¼ teaspoon of ground cardamom to the purée.

  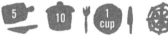

STONE FRUITS

4 stone fruits (such as peach, plum, nectarine), chopped, stones removed

1 Use a food processor or handheld blender to purée the fruit. Alternatively, put the chopped fruit in a small saucepan with 2 tablespoons of water. Cover and cook over low heat until tender.

2 Freeze in individual portions for up to 1 month or store in an airtight container in the fridge for 1 day.

SPICE IT UP:

Add ¼ teaspoon of ground cinnamon to the purée.

  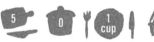

Meat purées

Chicken

100 g (3½ oz) boneless, skinless chicken breast, chopped

1 Put the chicken in a small saucepan with 625 ml (21½ fl oz/2½ cups) of water and bring to the boil. Reduce the heat to low and poach uncovered for 5 minutes or until the chicken is opaque and cooked through.

2 Use a food processor or handheld blender to purée with a little of the cooking liquid to reach the desired consistency.

3 Freeze in individual portions for up to 1 month or store in an airtight container in the fridge for 1 day.

SPICE IT UP:

Add ½ teaspoon of finely chopped fresh thyme leaves to the purée.

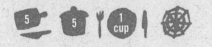

Beef, lamb, pork

Olive oil, for frying
100 g (3½ oz) minced (ground) beef, lamb or pork

1 Heat a little olive oil in a frying pan over medium–high heat. Add the meat and stir until browned and cooked through. Remove from the pan and set aside to cool.

2 Use a food processor or handheld blender to purée.

3 Freeze in individual portions for up to 1 month or store in an airtight container in the fridge for 1 day.

SPICE IT UP:

Add ½ teaspoon of minced garlic during cooking.

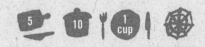

FISH

100 g (3½ oz) boneless, skinless pink
  salmon or firm white fish fillets

1 Steam the fish in a steaming basket
  until opaque and tender.

2 Use a food processor or handheld
  blender to purée with a little of
  the cooking liquid to reach the
  desired consistency.

3 Freeze in individual portions for up
  to 1 month or store in an airtight
  container in the fridge for 1 day.

SPICE IT UP:

*Add a pinch of finely grated lemon zest
to the purée.*

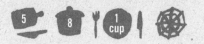

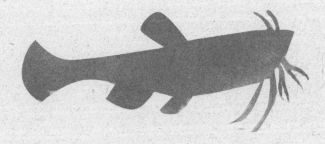

PAIR IT UP

These colourful purees will help ensure your baby is receiving a rainbow of nutrients. Simply add any protein/dairy or grain to any of these versatile bases for a well-rounded meal and textural change.

CARROT & APPLE

2 apples, peeled and coarsely chopped
1 carrot, peeled and coarsely chopped
¼ teaspoon finely grated fresh ginger

1 Steam the apples and carrot in a steaming basket until tender.

2 Use a food processor or handheld blender to purée with the ginger and a little of the cooking liquid to reach the desired consistency.

3 Freeze in individual portions for up to 1 month or store in an airtight container in the fridge for 1 day.

TIP:

Pairs well with chicken.

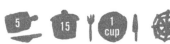

KALE & MANGO

8 g (¼ oz/¼ cup) kale ribbons (stalks removed, leaves sliced)
1 mango, peeled and coarsely chopped
½ teaspoon finely chopped fresh mint leaves

1 Steam the kale in a steaming basket until tender.

2 Use a food processor or handheld blender to purée with the mango and mint. Add a little cooking liquid to reach the desired consistency.

3 Freeze in individual portions for up to 1 month or store in an airtight container in the fridge for 1 day.

TIP:

Pairs well with fish.

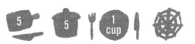

PUMPKIN & PARSNIP

150 g (5½ oz/1 cup) peeled, deseeded and
   chopped butternut pumpkin (squash)
1 parsnip, peeled and chopped
¼ teaspoon finely grated nutmeg
1 tablespoon olive oil

1 Preheat the oven to 180°C (350°F).
   Line a baking tray with baking paper.

2 Toss the pumpkin and parsnip with
   nutmeg and olive oil and scatter over
   the tray. Roast until caramelised and
   cooked through.

3 Transfer to a food processor or use
   a handheld blender to purée with a
   little cooled, boiled water to obtain
   the desired consistency.

4 Freeze in individual portions for up
   to 1 month or store in an airtight
   container in the fridge for 1 day.

TIP:

Pairs well with lamb.

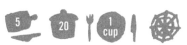

ZUCCHINI & APPLE

1 zucchini (courgette), peeled and chopped
2 apples, peeled, cored and chopped
½ teaspoon finely chopped fresh
   tarragon leaves

1 Steam the zucchini and apple in a
   steaming basket until tender.

2 Use a food processor or handheld
   blender to purée with the tarragon and
   a little of the cooking liquid to obtain
   the desired consistency.

3 Freeze in individual portions for up
   to 1 month or store in an airtight
   container in the fridge for up to 1 day.

TIP:

Pairs well with pork.

BANANA & BEETROOT

3 tablespoons peeled and chopped red
  beetroot (beet)
Olive oil, for drizzling
½ teaspoon finely chopped fresh sage leaves
2 bananas, peeled and chopped

1 Preheat the oven to 180°C (350°F).
   Line a baking tray with baking paper.

2 Toss the beetroot with a little olive oil
   and the sage and spread on the tray.
   Roast for 30 minutes or until tender.

3 Add the banana to the tray with
   the beetroot and return to the oven
   until the banana is caramelised and
   cooked through.

4 Transfer the beetroot and banana to
   a food processor or use a handheld
   blender to purée with a little cooled
   boiled water to obtain the desired
   consistency.

5 Freeze in individual portions for up
   to 1 month or store in the fridge for
   1 day.

TIP:

Pairs well with beef.

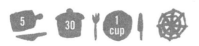

BLUEBERRY & PURPLE CARROT

2 purple carrots, peeled and chopped
80 g (2¾ oz/½ cup) blueberries

1 Steam the carrots in a steaming
   basket until tender.

2 Use a food processor or handheld
   blender to purée with the blueberries
   and a little of the cooking liquid to
   obtain the desired consistency.

3 Freeze in individual portions for up
   to 1 month or store in the fridge for
   1 day.

TIP:

Pairs well with chicken.

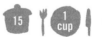

SWEET POTATO & APRICOT

1 large sweet potato, peeled and chopped
1 cupful of tinned apricot halves in natural juice
1/4 teaspoon ground cumin

1 Steam the sweet potato in a steaming basket until tender.

2 Use a food processor or handheld blender to purée with the apricots, cumin and a little cooking liquid to obtain the desired consistency.

3 Freeze in individual portions for up to 1 month or store in an airtight container in the fridge for 1 day.

TIP:

Pairs well with chicken.

  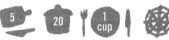

SPINACH & POTATO

2 large potatoes, peeled and coarsely chopped
Olive oil, to drizzle
1/2 teaspoon finely chopped fresh rosemary leaves
25 g (1 oz/1/2 cup) spinach leaves, destemmed
Greek-style yoghurt (optional)

1 Preheat the oven to 180°C (350°F). Line a baking tray with baking paper.

2 Toss the potato with a little olive oil and the rosemary leaves and spread on the tray. Roast for 30 minutes or until tender.

3 Transfer the potato to a food processor with the spinach (the spinach will wilt from the heat of the potato) or use a handheld blender to purée with a little yoghur, if using, to obtain the desired consistency.

4 Store in the fridge for up to 1 day. Not suitable for freezing if yoghurt has been added.

TIP:

Pairs well with chicken.

AVOCADO &
CUCUMBER

1 large avocado, peeled, stone removed
1 small cucumber, peeled, deseeded and
  coarsely chopped

1 Use a food processor or handheld
   blender to purée the avocado and
   cucumber with a little breastmilk or
   formula to the desired consistency.

2 Store in the fridge for up to 1 day.
   Not suitable for freezing.

TIP:

Pairs well with fish.

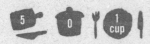

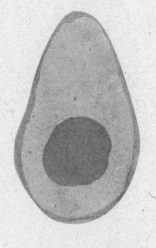

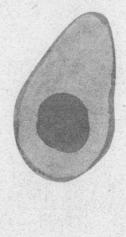

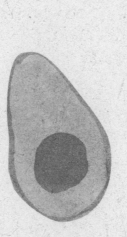

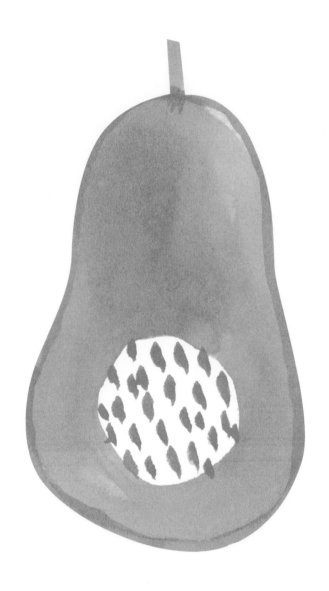

6-9 MONTHS

CHAPTER 6

The recipes in this chapter have been designed to help baby gently progress from starter purées to table foods that are packed with nutrition and flavour, providing a variety of different tastes, colours and textures. These unique, two-in-one, adult- and baby-friendly recipes take the guesswork out of preparing brain-boosting, nutritionally balanced meals for baby that can also be served as gourmet dinners for grown-ups.

A child's taste experiences during their first year can shape their preferences for years to come. Whether your baby partakes in family meals as purées or finger foods, it will help them develop their flavour and texture experiences, minimising future fussiness.

IRON BABIES

Solids introduced at around six months should start with foods that contain iron, essential for baby's brain, physical development and overall health. Iron-rich foods include:

HAEM IRON

Haem iron is found in animal foods. Red meat is the richest source.

- Beef; Lamb; Liver
- Pork; Chicken; Turkey
- Fish

NON-HAEM IRON

Non-haem iron is found mainly in plant foods and is not as easily absorbed by the body. It is still a very important source and is better absorbed if eaten with meat or foods high in vitamin C, such as oranges, strawberries, broccoli, tomatoes and capsicums (peppers).

- Iron-fortified infant cereal; Wheat biscuit breakfast cereal; Wholegrain cereals
- Cooked tofu; Legumes such as beans, chickpeas, lentils
- Eggs; Green leafy vegetables; Nuts and nut butters

6–9 MONTHS MEAL PLAN

	EARLY MORNING	MID MORNING	LUNCH	EVENING	DINNER	BEDTIME
DAY 1	Milk feed + Brain-boosting Brekkie (p93)	Milk feed	So Easy Salmon (p105)	Milk feed	Bambino's Baked Bolognese (p108)	Milk feed
DAY 2	Milk feed + Pear Porridge (p92)	Milk feed	Roast Vegetable Chips (p50)	Milk feed	Coconut Crumbed Fish with Mango Salsa (p103)	Milk feed
DAY 3	Milk feed + Mummy & Me Mango Porridge (p90)	Milk feed	Sweet Potato & Kale Bake (p104)	Milk feed	Roast Pork & Pears (p97)	Milk feed
DAY 4	Milk feed + boiled egg + toast fingers	Milk feed	Five-a-Day No-Crust Pie (p94)	Milk feed	Supercharged Shepherd's Pie (p98)	Milk feed
DAY 5	Milk feed + An Apple a Day (p91)	Milk feed	Supercharged Mash (p110)	Milk feed	Tiny Tots' Turmeric Chicken (p100)	Milk feed
DAY 6	Milk feed + avocado toast fingers	Milk feed	Busy Parents' Pumpkin Soup (p102)	Milk feed	First Fish Dish (p96)	Milk feed
DAY 7	Milk feed + Pear Porridge (p92)	Milk feed	Avocado Pesto Pasta (p112)	Milk feed	Lamb Shank Mash (p110)	Milk feed

MUMMY & ME MANGO PORRIDGE

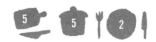

A nutrient-dense porridge for baby and delicious mango lassi for mum.

125 ml (4 fl oz/½ cup)
  coconut milk
100 g (3½ oz/1 cup) rolled
  oats (GF, if desired)
1 tablespoon chia seeds
160 g (5½ oz/½ cup)
  chopped fresh mango
Greek-style yoghurt, to serve

1 Combine the coconut milk with 250 ml (9 fl oz/
   1 cup) of water in a saucepan. Add the rolled
   oats and cook over medium heat for 5 minutes or
   until they have plumped up and softened, stirring
   constantly to prevent the porridge catching on the
   base of the pan. Add more water if needed.

2 Stir the chia seeds through the porridge, remove
   from the heat and set aside to cool.

3 When the chia seeds have plumped up, stir in the
   mango and a dollop of yoghurt.

FOR BABY:

Allow time to cool. Purée to desired consistency.

ALL GROWN UP:

*Add a little honey and yoghurt and whizz it up in
a blender to enjoy as a creamy mango lassi.*

SMART TIP
Chia seeds contain
plant-based omega–3
fatty acids and twice
the protein of any other
seed or grain.

AN APPLE A DAY

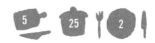

'An apple a day keeps the doctor away' is the old saying. This tasty treat will help boost baby's immune system.

4 medjool dates, pitted and finely chopped
200 g (7 oz/1 cup) quinoa, rinsed and drained
1 apple, peeled, cored and chopped
½ teaspoon ground linseed (flaxseed)
¼ teaspoon ground cinnamon
Small pinch grated nutmeg
Greek-style yoghurt, to serve

1 Put the dates and quinoa in a saucepan with 625 ml (21½ fl oz/2½ cups) of water over low heat. Simmer for 20 minutes or until tender, stirring occasionally to prevent sticking. To test tenderness, push the quinoa down on a wooden spoon – it should not have a hard centre.

2 Add the apple and cook for about 10 minutes until the apple is tender.

3 Set aside to cool. When you are ready to serve, mix in the linseed, nutmeg and cinnamon with a dollop of yoghurt.

FOR BABY:

Purée until it reaches the desired consistency. For younger babies, thin with a little cooled boiled water.

ALL GROWN UP:

Add some milk and honey if you like.

SMART TIP

Quinoa is high in fibre, folate, iron and protein.

PEAR PORRIDGE

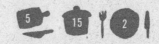

Wholesome and delicious, this pear porridge is sure to impress any little Goldilocks.

2 pears, peeled, cored and chopped
100 g (3½ oz/1 cup) rolled oats (GF, if desired)
¼ teaspoon ground cinnamon
1 teaspoon ground LSA meal (linseed, sunflower seeds, almond)

1 Put the pear in a saucepan with 625 ml (21½ fl oz/ 2½ cups) of water and bring to the boil. Reduce the heat and simmer for 10 minutes or until pear is soft.

2 Add the oats and cook for 5 minutes or until the porridge thickens. Stir in the cinnamon and LSA.

3 Remove from the heat and set aside for at least 5 minutes to cool and thicken.

FOR BABY:

Purée to desired consistency and stir in a little yoghurt.

ALL GROWN UP:

Add yoghurt and a drizzle of honey.

SMART TIP
Oats aid digestion and contain beta-glucans that boost the immune system.

BRAIN-BOOSTING BREKKIE

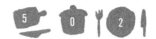

Give bub the best possible kick-start to the day with this breakfast.

115 g (4 oz/¾ cup) fresh blueberries

2 very ripe bananas, peeled

260 g (9¼ oz/1 cup) Greek-style yoghurt

230 g (8¼ oz/1 cup) fresh ricotta

2 teaspoons LSA meal (linseed, sunflower seed and almond)

¼ teaspoon ground cinnamon

1 Put the blueberries and bananas in a food processor and blend until smooth.

2 Add the yoghurt, ricotta, LSA and cinnamon and process until you obtain the desired consistency.

FOR BABY:

Purée to the desired consistency.

ALL GROWN UP:

Drizzle with honey, add milk and whizz into a breakfast smoothie.

SMART TIP

LSA meal (linseed, sunflower seed and almond) helps brain-processing speed while keeping the digestive system on track.

FIVE-A-DAY NO-CRUST PIE

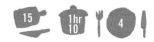

Getting your five serves of vegetables a day couldn't be easier with this simple-to-make pie.

½ butternut pumpkin (squash), peeled, deseeded and chopped
1 teaspoon ground nutmeg
170 ml (5½ fl oz) olive oil
1 large leek, washed and finely chopped
2 garlic cloves, crushed
25 g (1 oz/½ cup) spinach, coarsely chopped
6 eggs
150 g (5½ oz/1 cup) wholemeal self-raising flour (GF if desired)
100 g (3½ oz/1 cup) grated cheddar cheese
3 tablespoons marinated roasted capsicum (pepper) strips
230 g (8¼ oz/1 cup) fresh ricotta

1 Preheat the oven to 200°C (400°F). Grease a 23 cm (9 inch) round springform cake tin with butter.

2 Line a baking tray with baking paper and spread the pumpkin on it. Sprinkle with the nutmeg and drizzle with 2 tablespoons of the olive oil. Roast for about 30 minutes or until tender and golden.

3 Meanwhile, heat 1 tablespoon of the olive oil in a large frying pan over medium heat and fry the leek and garlic until translucent. Remove the pan from the heat and stir in the spinach until it is wilted and soft.

4 Whisk the eggs in a bowl and add the remaining olive oil and the flour, stirring until there are no lumps. Add the grated cheddar cheese.

5 Stir the pumpkin into the spinach mixture. Add the capsicum. Reduce the oven to 180°C (350°F).

6 Put half of the vegetable mixture into the cake tin, then pour half of the egg mixture on top. Give the tin a shake to ensure the egg mixture completely covers the vegetables. Add the remaining vegetable mixture and then the remaining egg mixture.

7   Spread the ricotta over the top, pressing it down
    a little so that it sinks into the egg mixture. Bake
    for 40 minutes until lightly golden and firm in the
    centre. Leave to stand in the tin for 5 minutes
    before removing the pie.

FOR BABY:

*Purée to desired consistency, or cut into small batons
as finger food.*

ALL GROWN UP:

*Season with salt and pepper and serve with a green
salad and balsamic dressing.*

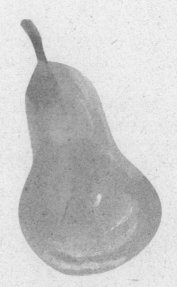

SMART TIP

*Ricotta is not only a good
source of calcium, it's high
in vitamin B12, which
plays a role in healthy
blood-cell function.*

FIRST FISH DISH

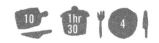

This creamy gratin is a wonderful first step into introducing baby to those essential omega–3s.

425 g (15 oz) tinned tuna in oil, drained
200 g (7 oz/1 cup) sweet corn kernels
25 g (1 oz/½ cup) spinach, finely chopped
20 g (¾ oz/1 cup) flat-leaf (Italian) parsley, finely chopped
1 leek, finely chopped
2 garlic cloves, crushed
2 teaspoons lemon zest
1 kg (2 lb 4 oz) royal blue potatoes, peeled and thinly sliced
200 g (7 oz/2 cups) grated parmesan or cheddar cheese
250 ml (9 fl oz/1 cup) pure (35% fat) cream

1 Preheat the oven to 180°C (350°F) and lightly grease a shallow ovenproof dish with a little butter.

2 Combine the tuna, corn, spinach, parsley, leek, garlic and lemon zest in a bowl.

3 Layer a quarter of the potato slices on the bottom of the ovenproof dish. Top with one-third of the tuna mixture and cover with 50 g (1¾ oz) of the cheese.

4 Repeat the layering, finishing with a potato layer. Press down firmly.

5 Pour the cream over the potato and spread the remaining cheese over the top. Cover the dish tightly with foil and bake for 1 hour.

6 Remove the foil and check that the potato is cooked through. Return to the oven and bake uncovered for 20–30 minutes until the top is light golden.

FOR BABY:

Purée to the desired consistency or cut into bite-size pieces for finger food.

ALL GROWN UP:

Season with salt and pepper and serve with green salad or coleslaw. You might like to scatter in a few capers.

SMART TIP
Tuna delivers critical omega–3 fatty acids that help regulate our inflammatory system. Our bodies cannot create these – they have to come from diet.

ROAST PORK & PEARS

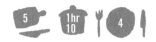

Sunday nights will never be the same again after you try this sumptuous dish.

2 tablespoons olive oil
4 pancetta slices, finely chopped
1 brown onion, diced
2 garlic cloves, crushed
230 g (8¼ oz/1½ cups) macadamia nuts, coarsely chopped
60 g (2¼ oz/1 cup) fresh breadcrumbs (GF if desired)
2 tablespoons finely chopped fresh sage leaves
1 egg, whisked
1.5 kg (3 lb 5 oz) boneless pork loin
5 pears, halved lengthways
2 tablespoons maple syrup
Sea salt, for rubbing
1 teaspoon fennel seeds, crushed

1 Preheat the oven to 220°C (425°F). Heat 1 tablespoon of the oil in a frying pan over medium heat. Add the pancetta, onion and garlic and cook until the onion is translucent, stirring constantly so the onion doesn't burn. Add the macadamias and cook until nuts are light golden. Set aside to cool.

2 Transfer the onion mixture to a bowl and stir in the breadcrumbs, sage and egg.

3 Lay the pork loin rind side up and pat dry with paper towel. Turn the pork over and flatten. Lay the stuffing in a line down the centre of the loin. Roll up the pork and tie with kitchen string at 3 cm (1¼ inch) intervals.

4 Place the pork in a roasting tin and arrange the pears around it. Drizzle the pears with maple syrup. Lightly score the pork rind and rub with sea salt and fennel seeds. Drizzle with the remaining olive oil and roast for 30 minutes.

5 Reduce the oven to 180°C (350°F) and roast for a further 40 minutes or until the pork is tender.

FOR BABY:

Make sure to remove any meat bones and the pips from the pears, then purée to desired consistency with some mashed potato and green beans.

ALL GROWN UP:

Season to taste and serve with mashed potato and green beans.

SMART TIP

Macadamia nuts are high in omega–3 fatty acids and might help increase the absorption of nutrients.

SUPERCHARGED SHEPHERD'S PIE

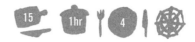

This family favourite has been given a smart makeover. Packed with veggies and flavour, this dish is bound to make you smile!

2 tablespoons extra virgin olive oil
2 onions, finely chopped
1 carrot, peeled and finely chopped
1 red capsicum (pepper), deseeded and finely chopped
2 garlic cloves, crushed
2 fresh thyme sprigs, leaves picked and finely chopped
1 sprig fresh rosemary, leaves picked and finely chopped
500 g (1 lb 2 oz) lean minced (ground) lamb

2 tablespoons wholemeal plain (all-purpose) flour (GF if desired)
3 tablespoons tomato paste
250 ml (9 fl oz/1 cup) salt-reduced chicken stock (GF if desired)
2 tablespoons Worcestershire sauce (GF if desired)
140 g (5 oz/1 cup) tinned four-bean mix, rinsed
140 g (5 oz/1 cup) frozen peas and corn mixture

TOPPING
2 large sweet potatoes (about 1 kg/2 lb 4 oz), peeled and coarsely chopped
2 tablespoons Greek-style yoghurt
1 tablespoon butter
A generous pinch of freshly grated nutmeg
50 g (1¾ oz/½ cup) grated parmesan cheese

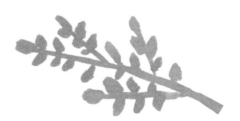

FOR BABY:

Purée to the desired consistency, or mash and roll into small balls for a soft finger-food option. Ensure the beans are well mashed before feeding baby.

ALL GROWN UP:

Season with salt and pepper and sprinkle with lemon zest for an extra kick.

1 Preheat the oven to 180°C (350°F).

2 To prepare the topping, put the sweet potato in a medium saucepan and cover with water. Boil over high heat for 15–20 minutes until tender, then drain and mash the potato with the yoghurt, butter and nutmeg until smooth. Set aside.

3 Meanwhile, heat the olive oil in a flameproof casserole dish and fry the onion, carrot and capsicum over medium heat for about 5 minutes until they start to soften. Add the garlic, thyme and rosemary and stir for a further minute. Stir in the lamb, breaking up any lumps, until browned. Pour the contents into a sieve to drain off any excess fat.

4 Return the lamb mixture to the casserole dish on the stovetop. Add the flour and cook, stirring, for a few minutes until the flour just starts to colour. Add the paste, stock, Worcestershire sauce, beans, peas and corn. Cover and simmer over low heat until the veggies have softened and the sauce has thickened.

5 Spread the topping on top of the lamb mixture, scatter with parmesan and bake for 30 minutes uncovered or until the topping starts to brown. Leave for at least 5 minutes to cool down before serving.

SMART TIP

Sweet potato boosts the immune system and, when paired with meat, its high vitamin C content helps baby's body absorb iron.

TINY TOTS' TURMERIC CHICKEN

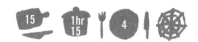

Don't miss out on your spicy favourites just because you are concerned mini-me might not enjoy them. Here we make a mild and slightly sweetened curry, taking out baby's dinner before we add the spicy curry paste.

1 tablespoon olive oil
700 g (1 lb 9 oz) skinless chicken breasts, thinly sliced
2 onions, finely chopped
150 g (5½ oz/1 cup) chopped butternut pumpkin (squash)
1 teaspoon ground turmeric
4 kaffir lime leaves
½ teaspoon ground cinnamon
3 star anise
375 ml (13 fl oz/1½ cups) coconut milk
125 ml (4 fl oz/½ cup) salt-reduced chicken stock (GF if desired)
60 g (2¼ oz/½ cup) sliced green beans
3 tablespoons tinned bamboo shoots, sliced
1 teaspoon coconut sugar
2 tablespoons salt-reduced soy sauce (GF if desired)
2 tablespoons fish sauce

CURRY PASTE
2 lemongrass stems
3 red Asian shallots
2 garlic cloves, crushed
10 cm (4 inch) piece fresh ginger, peeled and finely chopped
2 large chillies, deseeded

SMART TIP

Turmeric contains curcumin, which is an anti-inflammatory antioxidant that boosts brain function and protects brain health.

FOR BABY:

Purée the curry with some banana for a little sweetness.

ALL GROWN UP:

Serve with brown rice, basil leaves, cashew nuts and lime wedges. Season with salt and pepper.

1. To make the curry paste, whiz the lemongrass, shallots, garlic and ginger in a food processor or use a mortar and pestle to make a paste. Scrape into a small bowl and set aside.

2. Process the chillies in the food processor or use a mortar and pestle to make a red chilli paste to add to the adults' portions later.

3. Heat the oil in a heavy-based saucepan and brown the chicken. You don't want the chicken to stew, so you might need to do this in batches. Set aside.

4. Add the onions and pumpkin to the saucepan and cook for 5 minutes, until they start to soften. Add the curry paste and turmeric and stir for 3 minutes.

5. Return the chicken to the pan and stir well to coat in the paste. Add the kaffir lime leaves, cinnamon, star anise, coconut milk, stock, green beans, bamboo slices, sugar, soy sauce and fish sauce. Bring to the boil, then reduce to a very low simmer and cook for 45 minutes.

6. Remove the kaffir lime leaves and star anise and discard. Take out baby's serving and set aside. Add the red chilli paste and simmer for a further 15 minutes.

BUSY PARENTS' PUMPKIN SOUP

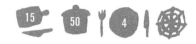

Cook up a big batch of this creamy soup and freeze it, ready to be reheated for a quick and nutritious weeknight dinner.

1.2 kg (2 lb 12 oz) butternut pumpkin (squash), peeled, deseeded and chopped
2 teaspoons dried sage
Olive oil, for drizzling
1 tablespoon butter
1 large leek, finely chopped
2 celery stalks, finely chopped
2 garlic cloves, crushed
115 g (4 oz/1 cup) walnuts, crushed to a powder
500 ml (17 fl oz/2 cups) salt-reduced chicken stock (GF if desired)
Pure (35% fat) cream, for serving

1 Preheat the oven to 180°C (350°F). Line a baking tray with baking paper.

2 Toss the pumpkin with sage and a little olive oil, coating it evenly. Spread over the tray and roast for 30 minutes until it starts to caramelise and develops a nice light golden colour.

3 Meanwhile, melt the butter in a large heavy-based saucepan over low heat. Add the leek and celery and fry gently until softened. Add the garlic and crushed walnuts and continue to cook for a further minute.

4 Transfer the roasted pumpkin to the saucepan with the leek mixture and stir before pouring in the chicken stock. Simmer over low heat for 20 minutes.

5 Use a handheld blender to purée the soup. Take out baby's portion.

6 Add the cream and process to a thinner consistency for adults.

SMART TIP

Walnuts contain neuroprotective compounds to support brain health.

FOR BABY:

Serve as a purée for a younger baby, or as soup with wholegrain toast fingers for an older baby.

ALL GROWN UP:

Top with chives and serve with crusty, seeded bread.

COCONUT CRUMBED FISH
WITH MANGO SALSA

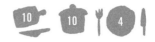

Mango has amazing antioxidant properties and loads of vitamins.

75 g (2¾ oz/½ cup)
   wholemeal plain
   (all-purpose) flour
   (GF if desired)
2 eggs
45 g (1½ oz/½ cup)
   desiccated coconut
60 g (2¼ oz/1 cup) fresh
   breadcrumbs
   (GF if desired)
Zest of 1 lemon
4 boneless white fish fillets,
   125 g (4½ oz) each
Olive oil, for cooking
1 lemon, quartered, to serve

MANGO SALSA
2 mangoes, peeled and
   chopped
2 tablespoons finely diced
   red onion
Zest and juice of 1 lime
1 avocado, diced
2 tablespoons fresh
   coriander (cilantro) leaves

1 To make the mango salsa, first reserve a little of
   the mango for baby. Combine the remaining mango
   with the other salsa ingredients in a bowl. Cover and
   refrigerate until needed.

2 Put the flour in a bowl. In a second bowl, whisk the
   eggs and in a third bowl mix the desiccated coconut
   with the breadcrumbs and lemon zest.

3 Dip each piece of fish into the flour, then the egg,
   followed by the coconut mixture. Ensure that each
   fillet is evenly coated with coconut crumb.

4 Heat a little olive oil in a heavy-based frying pan
   over medium heat. Fry the fish fillets for about
   4 minutes on each side, until cooked through.
   Do not overcrowd the pan.

FOR BABY:

*Purée the fish with the reserved mango or chop into
bite-size pieces for finger food. Add some cooked green
beans or Roast Vegetable Chips (page 50).*

ALL GROWN UP:

*Season with salt and pepper and serve with salsa and
roasted vegetable chips.*

SWEET POTATO & KALE BAKE

We've smartened up the traditional potato bake so that it's full of nutrient-rich veggies for bub and makes a sensational side dish for grown-ups.

300 ml (10 fl oz/1¼ cups) pure (35% fat) cream
1 garlic clove, peeled
A few grates of fresh nutmeg
3 thyme sprigs
Butter, for greasing
850 g (1 lb 14 oz) sweet potato, peeled and thinly sliced
50 g (2 oz/2 cups) kale ribbons (stalks removed, leaves sliced)
50 g (2 oz/½ cup) grated parmesan cheese

1 Preheat the oven to 180°C (350°F).

2 Put the cream, garlic clove, nutmeg and thyme sprigs into a saucepan and slowly bring to just below boiling point. Remove from the heat and set aside, allowing time for the flavour to infuse.

3 Grease a 27 cm (11 inch) round ovenproof dish with a little butter and place a layer of sweet potato slices across the base, followed by a layer of the kale. Repeat the layering process and finish with a layer of sweet potato.

4 Discard the garlic clove and thyme and pour the cream over the layered vegetables. Scatter the cheese over the top, cover with foil and bake for 1 hour. Remove the foil and bake for 15–20 minutes until light golden on top.

FOR BABY:

Purée to the desired consistency, adding a protein if desired.

ALL GROWN UP:

Season with salt and pepper and pair it with some lovely lamb chops.

SMART TIP
Kale is a powerful anti-inflammatory food, which helps protect against asthma, arthritis and autoimmune disorders.

SO EASY SALMON

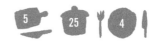

This delicious fish dish is so simple. All you have to do is spread the sauce over the salmon, stick it in the oven and voila! Dinner is ready.

260 g (9¼ oz/1 cup) Greek-style yoghurt
3 tablespoons finely chopped fresh dill
25 g (1 oz/½ cup) spinach, finely chopped
4 skinless, boneless salmon pieces, about 250 g (9 oz) each or 1 large fillet, pinbones removed
2 tablespoons dijon mustard
1 bunch young asparagus
Olive oil, for drizzling

1 Preheat the oven to 200°C (400°F). Lay the salmon skin-side down on a baking tray lined with baking paper. If using one whole piece of salmon, slice off a separate piece for baby.

2 Mix the yoghurt, dill and spinach together. Spread yoghurt mixture evenly over baby's piece of fish. Add the mustard to the remaining yoghurt mixture and stir. Spread evenly over the remaining salmon.

3 Line a separate baking tray with baking paper and spread the asparagus on it. Drizzle with a little olive oil and put it in the oven. After 5 minutes put the salmon in the oven with the asparagus and bake for 15–20 minutes until the fish is opaque.

FOR BABY:

Flaky salmon is a great finger food or you can purée it with some of the asparagus.

ALL GROWN UP:

Season with salt and pepper and add a squeeze of lemon.

SMART TIP

The 'good' fats in salmon are essential for brain development and improving memory.

ROAST VEGETABLE BAKED RISOTTO

Ever tried to stand at the stove and stir risotto with a wriggling baby on your hip? With this recipe you don't have to. And using pearl barley instead of arborio rice gives the risotto a wonderful nutty flavour.

3 tablespoons olive oil
2 carrots, peeled and chopped
2 red onions, peeled and cut into wedges
1 bunch baby beetroot (beets), peeled and
　　cut into small cubes
150 g (5½ oz/1 cup) peeled, deseeded and
　　diced butternut pumpkin (squash)
1 small head broccoli, cut into florets
200 g (7 oz/1 cup) pearl barley, rinsed and
　　drained (use quinoa as a GF alternative)
2 thyme sprigs, leaves picked
2 rosemary sprigs, leaves picked
2 tablespoons chopped basil, plus extra
　　leaves to serve
500 ml (17 fl oz/2 cups) salt-reduced
　　vegetable stock (GF if desired)
3 tablespoons crumbled feta cheese

SMART TIP

Barley contains lots of vitamins and minerals and the high fibre content helps baby stay regular.

1 Preheat the oven to 180°C (350°F). Pour the oil into a large roasting tin and heat it in the oven for 1 minute. Add the carrots, onion, beetroot, pumpkin and broccoli florets and stir. Return to the oven and roast for 15 minutes or until the vegetables start to soften. Remove from oven.

2 Add the barley, stirring well to coat the grains with the oil and mix through the vegetables. Add the herbs and stock, stirring gently.

3 Return the tin to the oven and cook for 40 minutes or until the barley is soft.

FOR BABY:

Purée to the desired consistency.

ALL GROWN UP:

Season with salt and pepper, then stir in the crumbled feta cheese and some extra basil leaves. Serve with a garden salad.

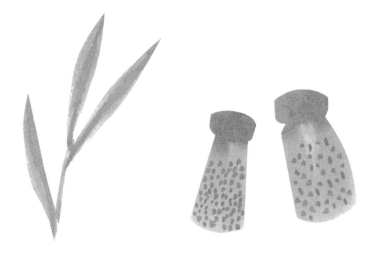

BAMBINO'S BAKED BOLOGNESE

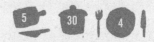

This recipe is a great way to ensure your bambino is receiving much-needed iron, essential for healthy brain development.

2 tablespoons olive oil
1 brown onion, finely chopped
90 g (3¼ oz/1 cup) coarsely chopped mushrooms
1 celery stalk, finely chopped
1 carrot, peeled and finely chopped
1 red capsicum (pepper), deseeded and finely chopped
1 garlic clove, crushed
1 teaspoon Italian herbs
300 g (10½ oz) vegetable-flavoured wholemeal spiral pasta (GF if desired)

250 g (9 oz) minced (ground) veal (or beef)
250 g (9 oz) minced (ground) pork (your butcher will mince the two meats together)
2 x 400 g (14 oz) tins chopped tomatoes
2 tablespoons tomato paste (concentrated purée)
125 ml (4 fl oz/½ cup) salt-reduced chicken stock (GF if desired)
460 g (1 lb/2 cups) soft ricotta cheese
100 g (3½ oz/1 cup) grated parmesan cheese

SMART TIP

Wholemeal pasta is an excellent source of complex carbohydrates, which provide glucose, important for fuelling the brain and muscles. It offers a slow release of energy and fibre.

FOR BABY:

Purée to the desired consistency.

ALL GROWN UP:

Season to taste and serve with green salad and balsamic dressing.

1 Preheat the oven to 220°C (425°F). Boil a large saucepan of water.

2 Heat the oil in a large heavy-based saucepan over medium heat. Sauté the onion, mushroom, celery, carrot and capsicum until softened. Add the garlic and Italian herbs and continue cooking for a further minute.

3 When the water is boiling, add the pasta and cook until just tender. Drain and set aside until needed.

4 Meanwhile, add the combined meat to the vegetables and cook, stirring constantly, until the meat is browned. Drain off excess fat if necessary.

5 Stir in the tomatoes, tomato paste and stock and simmer, uncovered, for a few minutes until the sauce thickens slightly. Remove from the heat.

6 Add the cooked pasta to the meat mixture and stir well. Transfer the mixture to an ovenproof dish.

7 Combine the ricotta and half the parmesan in a bowl and spread over the pasta mixture. Top with the remaining parmesan and bake for 10–15 minutes until lightly golden on top.

LAMB SHANK MASH

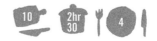

Slow-cooked and jammed with 'smart food' nourishment, these lamb shanks are the ideal family dinner. Don't shy away from using the anchovies in this recipe, they help to flavour the dish and benefit bub's brain development.

1 tablespoon fresh rosemary leaves
1 teaspoon ground coriander
1 teaspoon dried oregano
4 lamb shanks
2 tablespoons wholemeal plain (all-purpose) flour (GF if desired)
2 tablespoons olive oil
1 brown onion, chopped
1 celery stalk, sliced
2 garlic cloves, crushed
4 carrots, peeled and chopped
1 tablespoon balsamic vinegar
310 ml (10¾ fl oz/ 1¼ cups) salt-reduced chicken stock (GF if desired)
400 g (14 oz) tin chopped tomatoes
4 anchovy fillets
Juice of 1 lemon
Supercharged mash (page 49), to serve

1 Preheat the oven to 180°C (350°F).

2 Mix the rosemary, coriander and oregano in a bowl. Toss the lamb shanks in the herb mix, pressing it into the meat. Dust with flour until well coated, shaking off any excess.

3 In a large heavy-based flameproof casserole dish, fry the lamb shanks in the olive oil over high heat until well browned on all sides. Lift out onto a plate.

4 Lower the heat to medium and fry the onion, celery, garlic and carrots for a few minutes until softened.

5 Add the vinegar and boil for 30 seconds until syrupy. Add the stock, tomatoes, anchovies and lemon juice and bring to the boil. Return the lamb shanks to the casserole dish.

6 Cover and bake in the oven for 2 hours until falling off the bone. Uncover and bake for 10 minutes.

FOR BABY:

Purée the lamb meat with sauce and mash.

ALL GROWN UP:

Season with salt and pepper.

SMART TIP

Anchovies pack a nutritional punch – rich in omega–3s, magnesium, calcium and iron.

CHEAT'S GNOCCHI WITH CHERRY TOMATO SAUCE

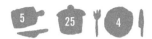

This is a fuss-free meal that does not lack flavour. The cherry tomato sauce delivers a natural sweetness that children just love.

2 tablespoons olive oil
1 brown onion, diced
1 garlic clove, crushed
500 g (1 lb 2 oz) cherry
 tomatoes, halved
500 g (1 lb 2 oz) packet
 fresh potato gnocchi
3 tablespoons chopped fresh
 basil leaves

1 Heat the olive oil in a heavy-based saucepan over medium heat. Fry the onion and garlic for about 5 minutes until softened.

2 Add the tomatoes, cover and simmer over low heat for 20 minutes, stirring occasionally. Gently push down on the tomatoes with the back of a spoon to help release the flavour.

3 Meanwhile, cook the gnocchi according to the packet directions.

4 Divide the gnocchi and sauce into serving portions and scatter with basil leaves.

FOR BABY:

Crush some walnuts and purée with the gnocchi until you obtain the desired consistency.

ALL GROWN UP:

Season with salt and pepper and top with crumbled goat's cheese and chopped walnuts.

SMART TIP

Tomatoes are rich in vitamin C, which helps improve the absorption of nutrients and vitamins.

AVOCADO PESTO PASTA

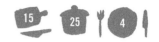

A deceptively light and summery pasta, combining a dizzying array of flavours and textures, this dish will be a firm family favourite in no time.

180 g (6¼ oz/2 cups) pasta, such as spirals or bowties
1 tablespoon olive oil
150 g (5½ oz/1 cup) grape tomatoes, quartered
Basil leaves, to serve
65 g (2½ oz/½ cup) crumbled feta cheese

AVOCADO, SPINACH & BASIL PESTO

25 g (1 oz/½ cup) baby spinach leaves
2 avocados, halved
3 tablespoons lemon juice
1 garlic clove, crushed
50 g (1¾ oz/1 cup) basil leaves
50 g (1¾ oz/¼ cup) pine nuts, toasted
3 tablespoons olive oil
25 g (1 oz/¼ cup) grated parmesan cheese

1 Cook the pasta according to the packet directions. Drain, reserving a little of the cooking water.

2 Meanwhile, make the pesto. Wilt the spinach leaves by pouring boiling water over them in a bowl and stirring well. Drain and squeeze dry.

3 Scoop the avocado flesh into a food processor and add the spinach, lemon juice, garlic, basil and pine nuts. Process until smooth, drizzling the oil in slowly. Finally, add the grated parmesan.

4 Heat the olive oil in a saucepan over medium heat. Add the tomatoes and toss quickly, then add the pasta, pesto to taste and enough of the reserved cooking water to make a sauce-like consistency. Gently toss until just combined.

5 Remove baby's portion before scattering with basil leaves and crumbled feta.

FOR BABY:

Purée to the desired consistency or cut into bite-size pieces to serve as finger food.

ALL GROWN UP:

Serve with a sprinkle of sea salt and freshly ground black pepper, and a squeeze of lemon. If you like a bit of heat then add some finely chopped chilli.

SMART TIP
Avocado is nutrient dense with more than 20 minerals and vitamins.

SPRING CHICKEN CASSEROLE

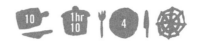

So easy you'll wonder why you haven't made this a hundred times already. So versatile you can add any vegetables and herbs you like.

1 tablespoon butter
4 skinless, boneless chicken thighs
1 leek, finely sliced
3 thyme sprigs, leaves picked
3 teaspoons salt-reduced chicken stock powder or 2 crushed stock cubes
2 tablespoons wholemeal plain (all-purpose) flour (GF if desired)
6 baby potatoes, quartered
2 carrots, peeled and coarsely chopped
50 g (1¾ oz/½ cup) frozen peas and corn mixture
1 tablespoon wholegrain mustard
Pure (35% fat) cream, to taste

1 Boil 750 ml (26 fl oz/3 cups) of water.

2 Melt the butter in a heavy-based saucepan over medium–high heat and brown the chicken. Do not overcrowd the pan. Remove chicken and set aside.

3 Add the leek and thyme to the saucepan and sauté until soft. Now add the stock powder and flour, stirring for a further minute.

4 Return the chicken to the pan and add the potatoes and carrots. Pour in the water and bring to a gentle simmer. Cover the pan and simmer for 30 minutes.

5 Add the peas, corn, mustard and cream and cook, uncovered, for a further 20 minutes, or until cooked through and the sauce has thickened.

FOR BABY:

Purée to the desired consistency.

ALL GROWN UP:

Season with salt and pepper and serve with crusty, wholegrain bread.

SMART TIP

Thyme is a natural immunity booster, packed with vitamins A and C. It has even been used to help alleviate coughing.

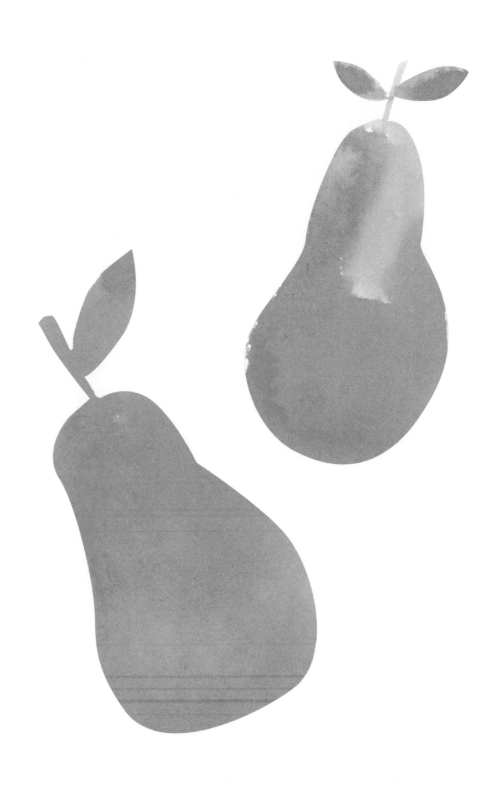

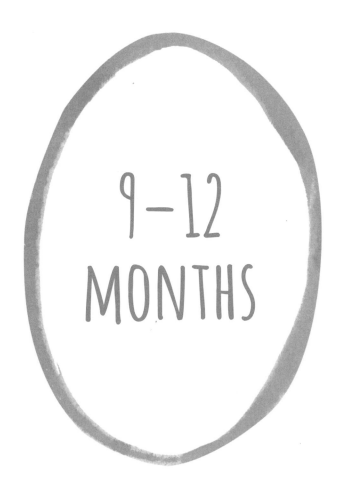

9–12
MONTHS

CHAPTER 7

9-12 MONTHS MEAL PLAN

	EARLY MORNING	MID MORNING	LUNCH	EVENING	DINNER	BEDTIME
DAY 1	Milk feed + Yoghurt Blueberry Pikelets (p120)	Milk feed	Green Pea Fritters (p127)	Milk feed	Slow Roast Chicken (p126)	Milk feed
DAY 2	Milk feed + Baked eggs 'n' beans (p121)	Milk feed	Cheesy Chomps (p138)	Milk feed	Stuffed Capsicum (p124)	Milk feed
DAY 3	Milk feed + Baby Bircher Muesli (p122)	Milk feed	Lemon Herb Fish Cakes (p136)	Milk feed	Mediterranean Bake (p131)	Milk feed
DAY 4	Milk feed + banana + boiled egg with toast	Milk feed	Mouthwatering Meatballs (p129)	Milk feed	When You Can't Be Stuffed (p134)	Milk feed
DAY 5	Milk feed + Purple Porridge (p123)	Milk feed	Quick Chicken Quinoa (p128)	Milk feed	Child-Friendly Chilli Con Carne (p130)	Milk feed
DAY 6	Milk feed + avocado toast fingers	Milk feed	Nanny's Chicken Noodle Soup (p132)	Milk feed	Friday Night Fish Fingers (p139)	Milk feed
DAY 7	Milk feed + Pear Porridge (p92)	Milk feed	Super Power Pesto with pasta (p135)	Milk feed	The Modern Mum's Sunday Roast (p141)	Milk feed

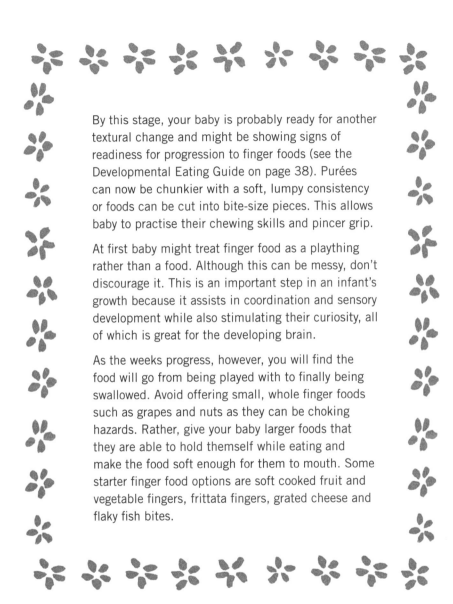

By this stage, your baby is probably ready for another textural change and might be showing signs of readiness for progression to finger foods (see the Developmental Eating Guide on page 38). Purées can now be chunkier with a soft, lumpy consistency or foods can be cut into bite-size pieces. This allows baby to practise their chewing skills and pincer grip.

At first baby might treat finger food as a plaything rather than a food. Although this can be messy, don't discourage it. This is an important step in an infant's growth because it assists in coordination and sensory development while also stimulating their curiosity, all of which is great for the developing brain.

As the weeks progress, however, you will find the food will go from being played with to finally being swallowed. Avoid offering small, whole finger foods such as grapes and nuts as they can be choking hazards. Rather, give your baby larger foods that they are able to hold themself while eating and make the food soft enough for them to mouth. Some starter finger food options are soft cooked fruit and vegetable fingers, frittata fingers, grated cheese and flaky fish bites.

FINGER FOOD BASICS

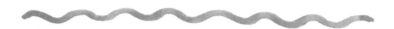

Prepare all fruit and vegetables by washing first. When cooking vegetables, use a steaming basket or steam in the microwave, rather than boiling – this will preserve as many nutrients as possible.

VEGETABLES

- Slice peeled carrot and pumpkin into sticks and steam using a steaming basket or in the microwave. Allow to cool before serving.

- Cut broccoli and cauliflower into florets. Ensure you leave as much of the stalk as possible so that baby has something to hold on to. Steam using a steaming basket or microwave in a bowl with a little water for approximately 2 minutes.

- Wedges made from potatoes, sweet potatoes or parsnips are all great finger foods. Try the Roast Vegetable Chips on page 50.

- Vegetables such as zucchini (courgettes) and carrots can be grated and eaten as they are or mixed with grated cheese.

- Technically avocado is a fruit, but most people consider it a vegetable. For a very messy, but extremely nutritious, snack slice avocado into segments.

FRUIT

- Ripe bananas make great finger food, but cut the banana into strips to guard against the possibility of choking.

- Cut mango into strips after removing the peel and seed.

- Slice soft plums, apricots or nectarines after the peel and stone have been removed.

- Apple can be grated. Alternatively, poach apples until softened and offer in segments.

- Pears can be poached and offered in segments. If a pear is very ripe, you can peel it and cut it into segments for baby without cooking.

MEAT

Cooked, cooled meat makes great finger food. Suitable meats include:

- Chopped chicken

- Chopped roast beef or lamb

- Small portions of cooked fish (remove any bones and skin)

TOAST

- Wholemeal toast fingers can be topped with mashed avocado, hummus, tahini, mashed banana, puréed vegetables, melted cheese (cool before offering), puréed fruit or mashed tuna with egg.

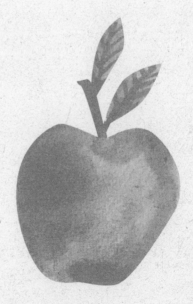

YOGHURT BLUEBERRY PIKELETS

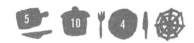

I don't think there is a kid in the world who doesn't love pikelets, and that includes all of us big kids too. Yoghurt, cinnamon and blueberries make this a nutritious breakfast or afternoon snack.

150 g (5½ oz/1 cup) plain (all-purpose) wholemeal flour (GF if desired)

2 teaspoons bicarbonate of soda (baking soda)

1 teaspoon ground cinnamon

2 eggs

390 g (14 oz/1½ cups) Greek-style yoghurt

2 teaspoons natural vanilla extract

155 g (5½ oz/1 cup) blueberries

Butter, for cooking

Maple syrup, to serve

1 Sift together the flour, bicarbonate of soda and cinnamon in a large bowl.

2 Add the eggs, yoghurt and vanilla and whisk to a smooth batter. If lumpy, strain through a sieve.

3 Fold in the blueberries, then set aside to rest for at least 10 minutes.

4 Melt 1 tablespoon of butter in a non-stick frying pan over low heat. Pour in a cupful of mix to make your pikelet. Cook until air bubbles start to appear on the surface. Flip the pikelet and cook until golden brown on both sides.

FOR BABY:

Cut up for finger food.

ALL GROWN UP:

Drizzle with maple syrup.

SMART TIP

An important probiotic, Greek-style yoghurt has more protein and less sugar than regular yoghurt.

BAKED EGGS 'N' BEANS

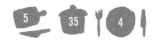

Traditionally spicy, this Middle Eastern breakfast gets a baby makeover without compromising on flavour or the wonderful health benefits of beans.

2 tablespoons olive oil
½ red onion, chopped
1 red capsicum (pepper),
   deseeded and chopped
400 g (14 oz/1½ cups)
   tinned cannellini beans,
   rinsed
300 g (10½ oz/1½ cups)
   chopped tomatoes
1 teaspoon paprika
½ teaspoon cumin
4 eggs
65 g (2½ oz/½ cup)
   crumbled feta cheese
30 g (1 oz/½ cup) chopped
   basil

1 Preheat the oven to 200°C (400°F). Heat the oil in a frying pan over medium heat and fry the onion and capsicum until caramelised. Add the cannellini beans, tomatoes and spices. Reduce the heat to low and simmer for 25 minutes. Set aside for 10 minutes to cool and then spoon the mixture into four ramekins or baking moulds.

2 Crack 1 egg into each mould. Crumble the feta evenly over the moulds and bake for 10 minutes. Finish with chopped basil.

FOR BABY:

Serve as it is for a textural change, or mash to the desired consistency.

ALL GROWN UP:

Enjoy with a piece of crusty, seeded bread.

SMART TIP
Eggs contain choline, which is an important nutrient for brain and nervous system function.

BABY BIRCHER MUESLI

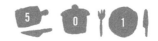

There's no reason baby has to miss out on this tasty treat just because they're small. Bircher muesli is full of nutritious fruit and yoghurt.

50 g (1¾ oz/½ cup) rolled oats (GF if desired)
185 ml (6 fl oz/¾ cup) milk
1 red apple
1 teaspoon ground cinnamon
3–4 fresh apricots, peeled, pitted and chopped
130 g (4½ oz/½ cup) Greek-style yoghurt
155 g (5½ oz/1 cup) blueberries

1 Before going to bed put the oats and milk in a glass or ceramic bowl and soak overnight in the fridge.

2 In the morning, grate the red apple and toss with the cinnamon. Mix in the apricots, yoghurt and the soaked oat mixture. Add the berries, then blend to the desired consistency, adding more milk if needed.

FOR BABY:

Purée to the desired consistency.

ALL GROWN UP:

Drizzle with some honey and blend to make a breakfast smoothie.

SMART TIP

Cinnamon can lower blood-sugar levels and reduce heart disease risk factors.

PURPLE PORRIDGE

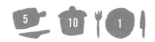

Frozen blueberries give this porridge an intense purple hue, making it fun for kids to eat as well as being super-nutritious and yummy.

100 g (3½ oz/1 cup) rolled oats (GF if desired)
1 teaspoon ground linseeds (flaxseeds) or chia seeds
1 banana, sliced
155 g (5½ oz/1 cup) frozen blueberries
50 g (1¾ oz/½ cup) almond meal
2 tablespoons Greek-style yoghurt

1 Gently cook the oats, linseed, banana and frozen blueberries with 625 ml (21 fl oz/2½ cups) of water in a saucepan over medium heat, simmering for around 6 minutes or until the oats are swelling up.

2 Remove from the heat and stir in the almond meal and yoghurt. Allow to cool before serving.

FOR BABY:

Purée to the desired consistency.

ALL GROWN UP:

Drizzle with some honey.

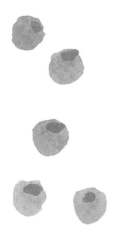

SMART TIP
Blueberries are believed to have the highest antioxidant capacity of all commonly consumed fruits and vegetables.

STUFFED CAPSICUM

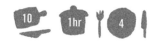

Transport dinnertime to Morocco with this simple yet exotic dish.

4 red capsicums (peppers)
2 tablespoons olive oil
1 large onion, finely chopped
200 g (7 oz) minced (ground) lamb or beef
200 g (7 oz/1 cup) brown basmati rice
90 g (3½ oz/½ cup) sultanas or currants
2 tablespoons dried mint
2½ teaspoons ground allspice
2 tablespoons lemon juice
80 g (3 oz/½ cup) sundried tomatoes, finely
   chopped
500 ml (17 fl oz/2 cups) salt-reduced
   chicken stock (GF if desired)
3 tablespoons pine nuts, toasted

YOGHURT DRESSING
130 g (4½ oz/½ cup) Greek-style yoghurt
2 tablespoons finely chopped fresh
   mint leaves
1 small garlic clove, crushed
Lemon juice

SMART TIP
Garlic is an
important
prebiotic food.

1 Preheat the oven to 200°C (400°F). Cut a 3 cm
(1 inch) wide circle around the stem of each
capsicum, remove the lids in one piece and set
aside. Remove and discard the seeds and pith.

2 Stand the capsicums in a deep-sided baking dish
and cover with foil. Bake for 30 minutes.

3 Meanwhile, heat a little of the olive oil in a large
frying pan over medium heat and cook the onion
until softened. Add the lamb or beef and cook until
browned. Add the rice and stir for 2–3 minutes,
making sure the rice is well coated.

4 Add the sultanas, mint, allspice, lemon juice and
sundried tomatoes to the pan. Stir well, then pour
in the stock. Bring to the boil then reduce the heat,
cover with a lid and gently simmer until the liquid
has been absorbed and the rice is tender.

5 Remove the capsicums from the oven and stuff the
lamb and rice mixture into the individual capsicums.
Pop the lids on and bake, uncovered, for a further
30 minutes. Five minutes before the end of the
cooking time, remove the lids and scatter pine nuts
evenly over the capsicums. Replace the lids and
return to the oven to finish cooking.

6 Meanwhile, make the yoghurt dressing in a small
bowl. Combine the yoghurt, mint and garlic and
adjust the flavour with lemon juice.

7 When the capsicums are cooked, remove them from
the oven and set aside for 5 minutes. Serve with a
spoonful of the yoghurt dressing.

SLOW ROAST CHICKEN

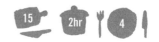

Cooked low and slow, this roast chook is divinely flavoursome and tender.
The Middle–Eastern rice stuffing gives it an exotic twist.

60 g (2¼ oz) butter
1 onion, finely chopped
1½ teaspoons ground
  allspice
75 g (2¾ oz/¼ cup) brown
  rice
170 ml (5½ fl oz/¾ cup)
  salt-reduced chicken
  stock (GF if desired)
35 g (1¼ oz/¼ cup) slivered
  almonds
40 g (1½ oz/¼ cup) pine
  nuts
85 g (3¼ oz/½ cup)
  sultanas
15 g (½ oz/½ cup) chopped
  flat-leaf (Italian) parsley
1 x 2.2 kg (5 lb) chicken
Olive oil, to drizzle

1 Preheat the oven to 180°C (350°F).

2 Melt a teaspoon of the butter in a frying pan and fry
   the onion. Stir in the allspice.

3 Add the rice to the pan and fry for a few minutes
   over medium–high heat.

4 Add the chicken stock and bring to the boil. Reduce
   the heat, cover and simmer for 20–25 minutes until
   the rice is cooked. Mix in the nuts, sultanas and
   2 tablespoons of the parsley and allow to cool.

5 Spoon the stuffing into the chicken cavity and put
   in a deep roasting tin. Mix the remaining butter with
   parsley in a bowl. Separate the chicken skin from
   breast and spread the butter under the skin. Truss
   the legs with kitchen string and drizzle a little olive
   oil over the chicken.

6 Roast for 2 hours or until the chicken is cooked
   through and the juices run clear when a skewer
   is poked into the thickest part of the thigh.

FOR BABY:

*Mash to the desired consistency or take some rice and
chopped chicken and form into balls for finger food.*

ALL GROWN UP:

*Season with salt and pepper and serve with roasted
vegetables or green salad.*

SMART TIP

*Allspice helps
to protect the
gastrointestinal
system and boost the
immune system.*

GREEN PEA FRITTERS

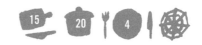

This is a light and refreshing meal that can be easily packed in a lunchbox, ready for a picnic play date.

140 g (5 oz/1 cup) frozen peas
125 ml (4 fl oz/½ cup) milk
2 eggs
15 g (½ oz) cornflour (cornstarch), GF if desired
100 g (3½ oz) plain (all-purpose) wholemeal flour (GF if desired)
½ teaspoon baking powder
50 g (1¾ oz/¼ cup) tinned corn kernels
150 g (5½ oz/1 cup) grated haloumi cheese
1 tablespoon finely chopped fresh mint
Olive oil, for frying

MINT YOGHURT

300 g (10½ oz) Greek-style yoghurt
10 g (½ oz) fresh mint
1 garlic clove, crushed
Squeeze of lemon juice

1   Boil the peas in a saucepan of water for 2 minutes. Drain and rinse under cold water. Mash or purée half the peas until smooth.

2   Whisk the milk, eggs, cornflour, flour, baking powder and puréed peas together in a bowl. Fold in the remaining peas, corn, haloumi and mint.

3   Heat some olive oil in a non-stick frying pan over medium heat. Drop tablespoons of the mixture into the pan. Cook fritters in batches, pressing down to flatten slightly, and fry for 1–2 minutes each side until golden brown. Drain the fritters on paper towel while you cook the remaining mixture.

4   To make the mint yoghurt, combine the yoghurt, mint and garlic and adjust the flavour with the lemon juice.

FOR BABY:

These make a great finger-food meal. Baby can enjoy dipping the fritters in mint yoghurt.

ALL GROWN UP:

Season with salt and pepper and serve with a dollop of mint yoghurt.

SMART TIP
Green peas are loaded with antioxidants and anti-inflammatory nutrients.

QUICK CHICKEN QUINOA

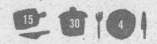

Superfood quinoa is bursting with proteins in this wonderfully light alternative to risotto.

500 g (17 fl oz/2 cups) salt-reduced chicken stock (GF if desired)

200 g (7 oz/1 cup) quinoa, rinsed well

Olive oil, for cooking

2 spring onions (scallions), finely chopped

2 skinless, boneless chicken thighs, sliced into strips

1 zucchini (courgette), finely chopped

1 tomato, finely chopped

65 g (2½ oz/½ cup) crumbled feta cheese

1 handful basil leaves, finely chopped

1 tablespoon lime juice

1 Bring the chicken stock and quinoa to the boil in a saucepan. Reduce the heat to low, cover and gently simmer for 10–12 minutes until the stock has been absorbed and the quinoa is cooked. The quinoa should be nice and fluffy.

2 Heat a little olive oil in a frying pan and fry the spring onions over medium heat until soft. After about 5 minutes, stir in the chicken strips and cook until the chicken is browned but still a little pink in the middle. Remove the chicken from the pan and set aside.

3 Add a little more olive oil to the pan and cook the zucchini and tomato until the zucchini is soft. Return the chicken to the pan and add the feta, basil and lime juice. Cook until the chicken is fully cooked and hot. Serve over hot quinoa.

FOR BABY:

Allow to cool and roll into soft balls for finger food, or mash to desired consistency.

ALL GROWN UP:

Season with salt and pepper.

SMART TIP

Zucchini contains vitamin C, a powerful antioxidant, which plays a big role in keeping the immune system healthy.

MOUTHWATERING MEATBALLS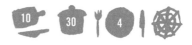

These yummy meatballs are packed full of veggies for bub and a flavour hit for the adults!

90 g (3¼ oz/1½ cups) fresh wholemeal breadcrumbs (GF if desired)
60 ml (2 fl oz/¼ cup) milk
600 g (1 lb 5 oz) minced (ground) pork
1 tablespoon finely chopped fresh coriander (cilantro) leaves
2 spring onions (scallions), finely chopped
2 tablespoons finely grated fresh ginger
80 g (2¾ oz/½ cup) peeled and grated carrot
70 g (2½ oz/½ cup) grated zucchini (courgette)
Olive oil, for drizzling
1 tablespoon sesame oil
3 tablespoons rice wine vinegar
170 ml (5½ fl oz/¾ cup) hoisin sauce (GF if desired)

1 Preheat the oven to 200°C (400°F). Line a baking tray with baking paper.

2 Combine the breadcrumbs and milk in a bowl and set aside for 5 minutes.

3 Add the pork, coriander, spring onion, ginger, carrot and zucchini to the breadcrumbs and mix well. Roll tablespoonfuls of meatball mixture into small balls.

4 Set baby's meatballs, evenly spaced, on the baking tray. Drizzle with a little olive oil and bake for 20–30 minutes until cooked through.

5 Heat the sesame oil in a frying pan over medium heat and cook the remaining meatballs for about 8 minutes until browned. Pour in 125 ml (4 fl oz/½ cup) of water, the rice wine vinegar and hoisin sauce and bring to a simmer. Give the pan a good shake until the meatballs are well coated. Cook for a further 10 minutes over low heat. Baby's meatballs should be ready at the same time the adults' meatballs are finished.

FOR BABY:

Serve the meatballs chopped with fingers of peeled and deseeded Lebanese cucumber.

ALL GROWN UP:

Season with salt and pepper and serve with a cucumber salad.

SMART TIP

Ginger is a potent antioxidant and anti-inflammatory agent.

CHILD-FRIENDLY CHILLI CON CARNE

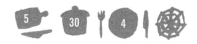

A child-friendly chilli con carne that is simple to make and packed full of healthy veggies and energy-rich ingredients.

1 tablespoon olive oil
1 small zucchini (courgette), grated
1 large carrot, peeled and grated
1 small red onion, diced
1 red capsicum (pepper), diced
1 teaspoon paprika
3 garlic cloves, crushed
½ teaspoon marjoram
1 teaspoon ground cumin
500 g (1 lb 2 oz) minced (ground) beef
2 tablespoons tomato paste
400 g (14 oz) tin diced tomatoes
300 ml (10½ fl oz) salt-reduced beef stock
400 g (14 oz) tin kidney beans, rinsed
400 g (14 oz) tin corn kernels
Juice of 1 lime, chilli powder or hot sauce, to taste

1 Heat the olive oil in a large frying pan over medium–high heat. Add the zucchini, carrot, onion and capsicum and cook for about 5 minutes until softened. Stir in the paprika, garlic, marjoram and cumin and mix well.

2 Add the beef mince and fry for 5 minutes or until the meat is browned. Add the tomato paste, beef stock, tomatoes, beans and corn and stir well. Leave to simmer for 20 minutes.

3 Remove baby's portion and then add the lime, chilli powder or hot sauce to taste.

FOR BABY:

Serve as it is for a textural change or purée to the desired consistency with a little sour cream and avocado. For finger food, roll into balls when cooled.

ALL GROWN UP:

Season to taste, add a little chilli or hot sauce and serve over brown rice, jacket potato or cheesy nachos.

SMART TIP
Beans are high in fibre and protein.

MEDITERRANEAN BAKE

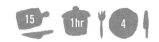

Like a cheesy baked risotto, this dish will have them queuing up for seconds... and even thirds!

Olive oil, for frying
1 eggplant (aubergine), diced
3 large carrots, peeled and chopped
3 celery stalks, thinly sliced
1 leek, finely chopped
3 garlic cloves, crushed
1 teaspoon tomato paste
500 g (1 lb 2 oz) tinned tuna in olive oil
110 g (3¾ oz/½ cup) marinated artichokes
180 g (6¼ oz/1 cup) risoni or 100 g (3½ oz/1 cup) small pasta (GF if desired)
375 ml (13 fl oz/1½ cups) salt-reduced vegetable stock (GF if desired)
2 tablespoons fresh thyme leaves
Zest of 1 lemon
65 g (2½ oz/½ cup) grated mozzarella cheese
2 tomatoes, sliced 1 cm (½ inch) thick
1 teaspoon dried oregano
50 g (1¾ oz/½ cup) grated parmesan cheese
3 tablespoons pine nuts
2 tablespoons coarsely chopped basil leaves

1 Preheat the oven to 180°C (350°F).

2 Pour a little olive oil into a large frying pan over medium heat and sauté the eggplant until it starts to turn golden brown. Remove from the pan and drain on paper towel.

3 Add the carrot, celery, leek and garlic to the pan and cook until soft. Add the tomato paste, tuna, artichokes and pasta and cook for 2 minutes.

4 Take the pan off the heat and add the stock, eggplant, thyme, lemon zest and mozzarella. Mix well and transfer to an ovenproof dish: 21 x 27 cm (8 x 11 inch) rectangle or 27 cm (11 inch) round.

5 Lay the tomato slices on top and sprinkle with oregano and parmesan. Bake for 45 minutes, sprinkle with pine nuts and bake for another 5 minutes. Scatter with fresh basil to serve.

FOR BABY:

Serve as it is for textural change or purée to the desired consistency (ensure pine nuts are crushed for baby).

ALL GROWN UP:

Season with salt and pepper and a squeeze of lemon juice.

SMART TIP

The phytonutrients in artichokes provide potent antioxidant benefit. The vitamin K content helps protect against cognitive diseases.

NANNY'S CHICKEN NOODLE SOUP

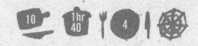

As ridiculously simple to make as it is nutritious, tasty and warming. This chicken noodle soup is the perfect base – add any extra vegetables you like.

1 x 2.2 kg (5 lb) chicken
1 teaspoon peeled and finely chopped
   fresh ginger
1 garlic clove, crushed
45 g (1½ oz/½ cup) thinly sliced mushrooms
¼ savoy cabbage, finely chopped
2 spring onions (scallions), finely chopped
45 g (1½ oz/½ cup) wholemeal pasta shapes
   or thin pasta broken into small pieces
   (GF if desired)
2 tablespoons soy sauce (GF if desired), plus
   extra to serve

STOCK

2 large onions, coarsely chopped
1 large celery stalk, coarsely chopped
1 large carrot, coarsely chopped
1 teaspoon fresh thyme leaves
½ bunch flat-leaf (Italian) parsley, leaves
   picked

SMART TIP
Celery has anti-inflammatory properties

FOR BABY:

Purée to the desired consistency or serve as it is and offer some toast fingers for dipping.

ALL GROWN UP:

Season with salt and pepper and add some finely chopped fresh chilli (if you like).

1 Put the chicken and the ingredients for the stock into a large saucepan or stockpot. Cover with water and bring to the boil. Reduce the heat to low and simmer for 90 minutes.

2 Remove the chicken from the stock and set aside to cool. Strain the stock, discarding the chopped vegetables, and return the liquid to the saucepan. When the chicken is cool enough to handle, remove the meat from the bones and return the meat to the stock, discarding the bones.

3 Add the ginger, garlic, mushrooms, cabbage, spring onion and pasta and return to medium–low heat. Simmer until pasta is cooked through and take out baby's portion. Add the soy sauce to the remainder for the adults.

WHEN YOU CAN'T BE STUFFED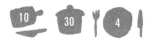

Celebrating the flavours of the Mediterranean, these stuffed eggplants are a satisfying meal in themselves.

2 eggplants (aubergines), halved lengthways
Olive oil, for cooking
½ red capsicum (pepper), deseeded and chopped
1 garlic clove, crushed
½ zucchini (courgette), chopped
140 g (5 oz/1 cup) tinned four bean mix, rinsed
3 teaspoons ready-made sundried tomato pesto
140 g (5 oz/1 cup) frozen mixed peas and corn
400 g (14 oz) tin tuna in olive oil, drained
2 tablespoons pure (35% fat) cream
125 g (4½ oz) grated haloumi or manchego cheese
3 teaspoons capers
Juice of 1 lemon

1 Preheat the oven to 160°C (315°F). Line a baking tray with baking paper.

2 Using a sharp knife, scoop out the inner flesh of the eggplants, leaving a shell about 1 cm (½ inch) thick. Lay the shells on the baking tray. Drizzle with a little olive oil and bake, covered with foil, for 25 minutes or until cooked through.

3 Meanwhile, heat a little olive oil in a frying pan over medium heat, sauté the capsicum, garlic and zucchini until soft. Add the beans, pesto, peas and corn, tuna and cream. Stir for 2 minutes until peas and corn are cooked through. Remove from the heat.

4 Take out baby's portion, fill their eggplant shell with the tuna mixture and top with grated cheese.

5 Add the capers and a squeeze of lemon juice to the remaining tuna mix. Fill the adults' eggplants and top with grated cheese.

6 Return the eggplants to the oven and bake, uncovered, until the cheese has melted.

FOR BABY:

Cut to a suitable size for baby.

ALL GROWN UP:

Season with salt and pepper and dig in.

SMART TIP

Eggplant contains nutrients that help to protect cell membranes from damage, particularly in the brain.

SUPER POWER PESTO

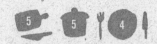

With a concentrated mix of powerful nutrients, this versatile pesto can flavour pasta, meats, vegetables or even seafood. Avocado, walnut oil and turmeric combine to make this an extra SMART addition to baby's diet.

1 large bunch mint, leaves picked
1 garlic clove, crushed
100 ml (3½ fl oz) walnut oil
40 g (1½ oz/¼ cup) pine nuts
25 g (1 oz/¼ cup) grated parmesan cheese
½ avocado
¼ teaspoon turmeric

1 Mix all the ingredients together in a food processor until a creamy paste forms.

SMART TIP

Mint promotes digestion and eases indigestion; great for gut health.

LEMON HERB FISH CAKES WITH AVOCADO CITRUS SAUCE

15 · 25 · 15 patties

Not your average fish patties, these lemon herb salmon cakes will have the fussiest of eaters lining up for more. The citrus sauce adds a silky flavour punch and bite-sized patties are perfect for little mouths.

1 large sweet potato, peeled and chopped

415 g (15 oz) tinned pink salmon

1 tablespoon finely chopped fresh flat-leaf (Italian) parsley

1 tablespoon lemon zest

2 spring onions (scallions), finely chopped

60 g (2½ oz/1 cup) wholemeal fresh breadcrumbs (GF if desired)

2 tablespoons finely chopped sweet gherkins or pickles

1 large egg, whisked

Olive oil, for cooking

AVOCADO CITRUS SAUCE

260 g (9¼ oz/1 cup) Greek-style yoghurt

2 tablespoons finely chopped fresh dill

1 teaspoon lemon juice

½ avocado, mashed

1 teaspoon garlic powder

1 Boil the sweet potato in a saucepan of water until tender. Drain and set aside.

2 Meanwhile, combine the avocado citrus sauce ingredients in a bowl and keep in the fridge.

3 Drain the salmon and mash with a fork in a large bowl. Add the parsley, lemon zest, spring onions, cold mashed sweet potato, breadcrumbs, gherkins and egg. Mix everything together. Form the mixture into small round bite-size patties.

4 Heat some olive oil in a non-stick frying pan over medium heat. Place the salmon patties in the pan and cook for 2–4 minutes on each side until they are heated through and have a golden crust.

FOR BABY:

Serve as finger food with avocado citrus sauce for dipping.

ALL GROWN UP:

Season with salt and pepper and serve with avocado citrus sauce and a green salad.

SMART TIP

Dill aids digestion and offers anti-inflammatory and antiviral properties.

GREEK LEMON CHICKEN

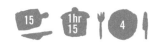

This dish doesn't just taste great, it fills the house with delicious aromas, defying anyone to say they aren't hungry. It's impossible to resist!

1.5 kg (3 lb 5 oz) chicken drumsticks
2 red onions, quartered
15 black olives, pitted
3 tomatoes, quartered
275 g (10 oz) marinated artichokes
400 g (14 oz) tin four-bean mix, rinsed
3 royal blue potatoes, quartered
Juice of ½ lemon
2 tablespoons olive oil, plus extra for drizzling
3 garlic cloves, crushed
270 ml (9½ fl oz) salt-reduced chicken stock (GF if desired)
3 thyme sprigs, leaves picked
2 tablespoons almond flakes, toasted, to serve

1 Preheat the oven to 180°C (350°F). Put the chicken drumsticks, onion, olives, tomato, artichokes, beans and potatoes in a large ovenproof dish.

2 Combine the lemon juice, olive oil, garlic and chicken stock in a jug. Pour over the chicken and vegetables in the dish.

3 Scatter the thyme leaves over the top and drizzle with a little oil. Bake uncovered for 1 hour. If not quite browned on top, cook for a further 30 minutes. Scatter with almond flakes to serve.

FOR BABY:

Cut up for finger food with some steamed broccoli florets or mash to desired consistency.

ALL GROWN UP:

Season with salt and pepper and enjoy with steamed broccoli.

SMART TIP
Lemon boosts the immune system and aids the absorption of iron.

CHEESY CHOMPS

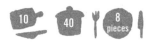

Perfect for a play date, these vegetable–rice fingers will be the stuff of legend at playgroup.

1 tablespoon olive oil
1 leek, finely chopped
1 garlic clove, crushed
1 zucchini (courgette), finely grated
1 carrot, finely grated
1 red capsicum (pepper), finely chopped
200 g (7 oz/1 cup) tinned corn kernels
2 eggs, whisked
150 g (5½ oz/1½ cups) grated cheddar cheese
280 g (10 oz/1½ cups) cooked brown rice

1 Preheat the oven to 180°C (350°F). Lightly grease a baking tin.

2 In a saucepan, heat the oil over medium heat and fry the leek, garlic and all the vegetables until softened. Remove from the heat and set aside to cool for 10 minutes.

3 In a bowl combine the eggs, half the cheese, the rice and the vegetable mixture.

4 Put the mixture into the baking tin. Scatter with the remaining cheese and bake for 30–35 minutes until golden. Cut into batons.

FOR BABY:

Serve as batons for a great finger-food option.

ALL GROWN UP:

Serve with a garden salad.

SMART TIP

Zucchini is rich in vitamin C, omega–3s, vitamin B, fibre and calcium.

FRIDAY NIGHT FISH FINGERS

These finger-licking fish fingers are much healthier than shop-bought versions.
Serve with minty mashed peas.

4 x 200 g (7 oz) skinless,
boneless snapper fillets,
or other firm white-fleshed
fish
50 g (1¾ oz/½ cup) almond
meal
50 g (1¾ oz/½ cup) finely
grated parmesan cheese
2 tablespoons chopped
fresh dill
2 tablespoons olive oil

YOGHURT DIP
260 g (9¼ oz/1 cup) Greek-
style yoghurt
2 tablespoons finely
chopped dill
1 teaspoon lemon juice
½ avocado, mashed
1 teaspoon garlic powder

1 Preheat the oven to 220°C (425°F). Line a baking
tray with baking paper.

2 Combine the yoghurt dip ingredients in a small bowl
and keep in the fridge until ready to use.

3 Cut the fish fillets into fingers. In a bowl, combine
the almond meal, parmesan, dill and olive oil.
Crumble the mix with your fingers to create a coating
for the fish. Crumb fish fingers individually, pressing
the coating onto the fish. Lay the fish fingers on the
baking tray and put in the fridge for 10 minutes.

4 Bake the fish fingers for 12 minutes or until the fish
is opaque and crumb is golden.

FOR BABY:

*Baby will enjoy dipping the fish fingers into
the yoghurt dip.*

ALL GROWN UP:

Serve with extra lemon wedges.
Season with salt and pepper.

SMART TIP

Almonds are loaded
with antioxidants and
almond meal is a
safe way for baby
to eat them.

BUB'S OSSO BUCO

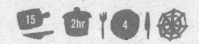

Osso buco brings back memories of winter dinners with the whole family, the hearty food warming us from the inside. Start making early memories with this dish – it can be slow-cooked during the day and served with some lovely Supercharged Mash (page 49).

2 tablespoons olive oil
4 pieces of veal shin with the bone in
Wholemeal plain (all-purpose) flour, for dusting (GF if desired)
120 g (4¼ oz) unsalted butter
1 tablespoon chopped fresh sage
1 garlic clove, crushed
2 brown onions, chopped
1 carrot, peeled and chopped
1 celery stalk, chopped
270 ml (9½ fl oz) salt-reduced chicken stock (GF if desired)
4 tablespoons verjuice

GREMOLATA
Zest of 1 lemon
3 tablespoons chopped flat-leaf (Italian) parsley
2 garlic cloves, crushed

1 Heat the oil in a heavy-based saucepan that is large enough to hold the meat in a single layer. Dust the meat with flour and fry until browned on both sides. Do not overcrowd the pan (you might need to brown the meat in batches). Remove the meat from the pan and set aside.

2 Add the butter, sage, garlic, onion, carrot and celery and fry for a few minutes. Add the chicken stock and verjuice and bring to the boil. Turn the heat down to a gentle simmer and return the meat to the pan, ensuring it is covered by stock. Cover with a lid.

3 Turn the meat every 30 minutes for a total of 2 hours. Lift the lid and stir in the gremolata mix.

4 Remove from the heat and set aside for 10 minutes before serving, spooning the sauce over the meat.

FOR BABY:

Remove the meat from the bone and purée to desired consistency with some Supercharged Mash.

ALL GROWN UP:

Season with salt and pepper and serve with Supercharged Mash.

SMART TIP
Sage aids cognitive function and is high in antioxidants to protect from free radicals.

THE MODERN MUM'S SUNDAY ROAST

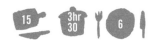

It doesn't get better than a good old-fashioned roast with a nutritious twist! This pulled Persian lamb is delicious with a refreshing cucumber salad, or serve with your choice of roasted veggies.

4 tablespoons pomegranate molasses
2 garlic cloves, crushed
1 teaspoon ground cumin
1 tablespoon olive oil
Juice of 1 lemon
½ teaspoon dried mint
1 onion, coarsely chopped
1.5 kg (3 lb 5 oz) lamb shoulder

CUCUMBER SALAD
3 large cucumbers
2 tablespoons Greek-style yoghurt
1 tablespoon vinegar
1 tablespoon olive oil
1 teaspoon coconut sugar
1 tablespoon dried mint

1 Preheat the oven to 160°C (315°F). Mix the molasses, garlic, cumin, olive oil, lemon juice and mint in a small bowl. Spread the chopped onion evenly over the base of a deep roasting tin. Lay the lamb on top of the onions and pour the molasses over the top. Pour about 200 ml (7 fl oz) of water into the tin.

2 Cover tightly with foil and roast, undisturbed, for 3 hours. Remove the foil and roast for a further 30 minutes.

3 Meanwhile, for the salad, deseed and chop the cucumbers. Mix together with the remaining ingredients and season with salt to taste.

4 Allow the lamb to rest after cooking for 10 minutes. Carve and serve with cucumber salad.

FOR BABY:

Chop up for finger food or purée with roast vegetables.

ALL GROWN UP:

Season with salt and pepper and serve with the cucumber salad or some roasted vegetables.

SMART TIP
Pomegranate is loaded with vitamins, minerals, fibre and antioxidants.

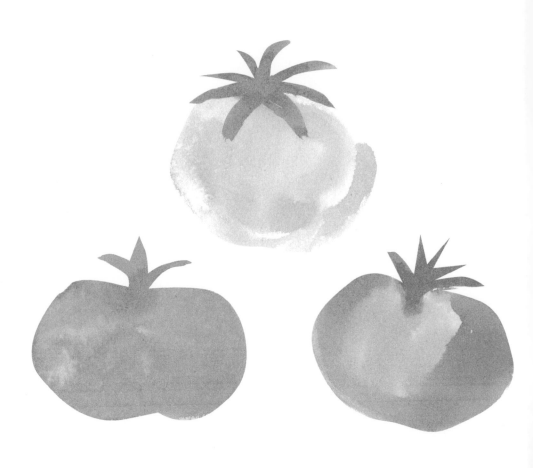

TODDLER
TIME

CHAPTER 8

Just when you think you've nailed this parenthood thing and start to visualise yourself sipping pina coladas in the Caribbean... BOOM! Toddlerhood arrives, and overnight your angelic baby has turned into a pint-sized, tantrum-throwing food critic who rejects every meal you put in front of them. What happened? You followed the advice, did everything you thought you were supposed to, but now you're wondering how soon they'll be old enough to send to boarding school. What went wrong?

Absolutely nothing. It is actually very common for even the most adventurous eaters to experience some food fussiness at least once during their childhood. Generally, it begins around the 18-month mark. Around this age, toddlers lose some of their appetite because their growth rate is not as rapid as it has been. They're also quite mobile and very curious, so they prefer to explore the world around them rather than waste time eating.

Teething issues such as the painful eruption of their first molars can also affect their desire for food, leading them to reject chewy foods and opt for liquids or soft food instead. It's also possible that a bit of 'food neophobia' (fear of new foods) has started to surface, and this too is quite common as your child learns to recognise and associate colour, texture and shape with the taste of different foods.

Don't despair: there are a few things you can do to help them past this stage. Below is a list of strategies to try:

- **START OUTSIDE THE KITCHEN.** From smelling rosemary plants while out on a walk, to watering the herb garden, use every opportunity to allow your child to interact with food in a fun, positive and stimulating way. Getting them outdoors to help plant veggies and painting or playing games with food is a great sensory way to introduce and talk about new foods. Although it might be messy, don't discourage this. Forget all the times your parents told you not to play with your food – just grab the wipes and let your child go for it. It's an important step in helping expand taste preferences, coordination, sensory and brain development.

- **GET THEM INVOLVED.** Involve your child in the mealtime ritual. Get them in the kitchen to help prepare or watch you cook. Toddlers love duties, so giving them responsibilities such as helping to cook, setting the table, choosing music to cook with, picking herbs, shopping, and so on all helps them feel a part of something. Most children will eat or at least try a taste of a meal they have helped to create.

- **FAMILIARITY.** This is one time familiarity does not breed contempt. The more familiar your child is with a food, the more likely they will be to accept it, so keep offering foods they've rejected. In most cases, repeatedly offering and encouraging them to taste previously rejected foods will eventually lead to your child tolerating and enjoying them. It may take 10–20 tastes before they accept a new food, so don't give up too early.

- **BABY SEE, BABY DO.** Children imitate our good and bad habits so keep eating those veggies and make sure your child eats with you as a family. The more they see you eat and enjoy a variety of foods, the more they will be inclined to accept the same variety.

- **NO REWARDS.** Offering rewards might work in the short-term, but this tactic tends to teach children that being a difficult eater gets them attention and something nice. Although your child might finish their plate of peas, in the long term they are less likely to enjoy peas and more likely to manipulate you at mealtimes. Instead of offering a reward, give them a choice between two nutritious options. Toddlers love to exert independence, so being able to make a choice between something like peas or corn, for example, gives them a sense of independence.

- **PRAISE.** Praise their efforts to try new foods. It helps develop a positive association and gets you one babystep closer to actually eating the new foods.

- **POSITIVE MEALTIMES.** Be patient and nurturing with your child when trying new foods. Offering a new food alongside a favourite food and asking them to try a small amount helps to keep mealtimes a positive experience while also taking the pressure off your child.

- **EDUCATE.** Children love to learn. Mealtimes provide the perfect opportunity to discuss where their food comes from in a fun and informative way. Get creative and turn food into magical stories that stimulate their curiosity. You could create funny faces or animals with their food or make tasting plates from different cuisines to bring a sense of fun and add to the magic of mealtime.

● SNACKS. Nutritious, balanced snacks can be key in preventing erratic eating behaviour. Offering your toddler nutritious snacks doesn't just prevent them becoming 'hangry' (hungry–angry) in between meals, but it is a great way to build more nutrients into their daily diet. Toddlers are on the move nonstop, and require plenty of opportunities to fuel their energy. Keeping in mind that their tummies are still quite small, it is a good idea to offer three meals and two snacks a day.

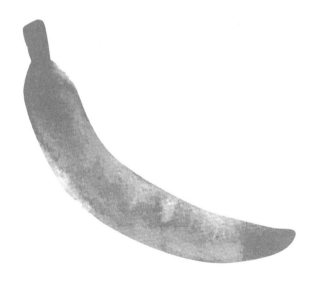

TODDLER MEAL PLAN

	BREAKFAST	SNACK	LUNCH	SNACK	DINNER
DAY 1	Homemade Baked Beans (p148) + Wholemeal toast fingers	Savoury Scrolls (p162)	Pumpkin & Feta Rolls (p155)	Blueberry Frozen Yoghurt (p157)	Pasta Perfection (p167)
DAY 2	Quick Quiches (p149)	Holy Guacamole (p161) + carrot sticks	Mac 'n' Cheese Cups (p159)	Fruit	Pancakes For Dinner (p164)
DAY 3	Banana Smoothie (p150)	Fruit	Smoked Salmon Finger Sandwiches (p153)	Quick Quiches (p149)	Five-Minute Fried Rice (p165)
DAY 4	Egg Rolls (p152)	Crushed almonds + fruit + yoghurt	Dumplings (p154)	Veggie sticks	Baked Carbonara (p171)
DAY 5	Blueberry Smoothie (p150)	Fruity Fingers (p158)	Veggie Slice (p160)	Savoury Scrolls (p162)	Chicken Schnitzel Strips (p166)
DAY 6	Baby's Bircher Muesli (p122)	Veggie sticks + hummus	Chicken Waldorf Finger Sandwiches (p153)	Fruit	Better For You Bangers & Mash (p170)
DAY 7	Wholesome Banana Bread (p151)	Crushed walnuts + yoghurt	Sushi Balls (p156)	Boiled egg + fruit	Friday Night Pizza (p168)

HOMEMADE BAKED BEANS

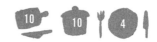

Forget the salt- and sugar-laden ready-made tinned variety: these wholesome beans are the bomb!

1 tablespoon olive oil
1 red onion, finely chopped
1 tablespoon tomato paste
400 g (14 oz) tin crushed
   tomatoes
1 tablespoon Worcestershire
   sauce
1 teaspoon maple syrup
2 x 400 g (14 oz) tins four-
   bean mix, rinsed

1 Heat the oil in a small saucepan over medium heat. Add the onion and cook for 3–4 minutes until soft.

2 Reduce the heat to low and stir in the tomato paste. Add the tomatoes, Worcestershire sauce, maple syrup and bean mix.

3 Stir well and simmer for 5 minutes until the sauce thickens.

FOR TODDLER:

Serve with some wholemeal toast fingers.

ALL GROWN UP:

Add some ham off the bone, dijon mustard and smoked paprika for an extra kick.

SMART TIP
Aside from protein, fibre and complex carbohydrates, beans contain numerous antioxidants, vitamins and minerals.

QUICK QUICHES

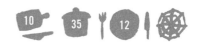

Quiches are a great way to use up leftover vegetables. Offer a variety of fillings so your toddler can experience different flavours and nutrients. These crustless quiches make for a fast and nutritious breakfast or lunchbox item.

2 tablespoons butter
1 onion, finely chopped
1 bunch asparagus, finely chopped
160 g (5½ oz) additive-free ham, finely chopped
4 eggs
2 egg yolks
500 ml (17 fl oz/2 cups) pure (35% fat) cream
100 g (3½ oz/1 cup) grated cheddar cheese

1   Preheat the oven to 180°C (350°F). Lightly grease a 12-hole muffin tin.

2   Melt the butter in a small frying pan over medium heat and sauté the onion and asparagus until soft. Stir in the ham.

3   In a bowl, whisk together the eggs, egg yolks and cream.

4   Spoon the asparagus mixture into the muffin holes and top with the cheese. Pour egg mixture into each muffin hole until it is nearly full.

5   Bake for 25–30 minutes or until the egg mixture is firm to the touch and golden on top. Cool for 5 minutes and then remove from the tin.

FOR TODDLER:

Serve as a great breakfast-on-the-go option or lunchbox item.

ALL GROWN UP:

Serve with a crisp green salad and season with salt and pepper.

SMART TIP

Asparagus is packed with nutrients that have antioxidant and anti-inflammatory properties.

SMART SMOOTHIE BASE

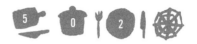

A smoothie can be a wonderful vehicle for packing in the nutrition. All you need is a 'smart' base and you can add any fruits or vegetables you like.

250 ml (9 fl oz/1 cup) milk
130 g (4½ oz/½ cup)
  Greek-style yoghurt
1 teaspoon honey or maple
  syrup or agave syrup
1 teaspoon LSA meal
  (linseed, sunflower seed
  and almond)
1 small banana
1 cupful chopped fruit or
  vegetables, such
  as blueberries
Ice cubes (optional)

1 Combine all the ingredients in a blender and process until you obtain the desired consistency. Serve.

FOR TODDLER:

Let your toddler choose their smoothie additions to create a little fun and a sense of responsibility.

ALL GROWN UP:

Even if you have a preferred smoothie flavour, make sure you change it regularly for nutritional variety.

SMART TIP
Greek-style yoghurt has less sugar than most other yoghurts. Yoghurt is a great source of probiotics and calcium.

WHOLESOME BANANA BREAD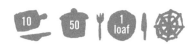

Bake the night before for a grab 'n' go breakfast option.

260 g (9¼ oz/1¾ cups) wholemeal plain (all-purpose) flour (GF if desired)

1 teaspoon ground cinnamon, plus extra to sprinkle

1 teaspoon baking powder

1 teaspoon bicarbonate of soda (baking soda)

2 eggs

125 ml (4 fl oz/½ cup) melted coconut oil or olive oil

4 tablespoons honey, maple syrup or rice malt syrup

65 g (2½ oz/¼ cup) Greek-style yoghurt

1 teaspoon natural vanilla extract

4 ripe bananas, mashed, plus a few extra slices for decorating

60 g (2¼ oz/½ cup) crushed walnuts

1 Preheat the oven to 180°C (350°F). Lightly grease a 10 x 20 cm (4 x 8 inch) loaf tin.

2 Mix together the flour, cinnamon, baking powder and bicarbonate of soda.

3 In a large bowl whisk the eggs, coconut oil, honey, yoghurt and vanilla for a few minutes. Stir in the mashed banana, flour mixture and crushed walnuts.

4 Pour the mixture into the loaf tin. Top with banana slices and sprinkle with a little extra cinnamon. Bake for 45–50 minutes until cooked through.

FOR TODDLER:

If you need a nut-free loaf for the lunchbox, just leave out the walnuts.

ALL GROWN UP:

Spread with a little butter and put your feet up.

SMART TIP

Bananas contain nutrients that help moderate blood-sugar levels.

EGG ROLLS

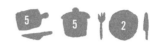

Toddlers love small things and these little egg rolls make for a fun finger-food breakfast or lunch item. We have used salmon for a hit of omega–3; however, you can pick your fillings as you please.

120 g (4¼ oz/½ cup) cream cheese, softened
1 teaspoon finely chopped fresh dill
100 g (3½ oz) smoked salmon, finely chopped
3 eggs, whisked
1 tablespoon pure (35% fat) cream
Butter, for cooking

1 In a small bowl, mix together the cream cheese, dill and salmon and set aside.

2 Whisk the eggs and cream together in a small bowl. Heat a small non-stick frying pan with a little butter over low heat.

3 Pour enough egg mixture into the pan to create a thin pancake.

4 Wait for the egg to lightly brown and then flip it over to cook on the other side.

5 Repeat until the mixture runs out. Lay the pancakes on a chopping board and spread with the salmon mixture. Roll them up into cigar shapes and then cut into rounds.

FOR TODDLER:

Serve as finger food or use the egg pancakes as a base for trying out all sorts of different fillings.

ALL GROWN UP:

Great finger food for a morning-tea play date.

SMART TIP
Eggs are highly nutritious, containing a little bit of almost every nutrient we need.

TODDLER TAPAS

~~~~~~~~~~~~~~~~~~~~~~~~~~

During this developmental stage you may find that your toddler is more attracted to a variety of little foods in one sitting. The 'tapas' technique of several small food items keeps it fun, nutritious and continues to build their taste exposure.

The following foods are designed to be enjoyed as part of a tapas-style lunch or snack. For a well-balanced meal, serve them alongside some chopped fresh fruit, vegetables, dip, chopped nuts, cheese, yoghurt or a protein of your choice.

FINGER SANDWICH FILLINGS

Don't get stuck in a rut with the same old sandwich fillings; offer these up instead.

HAM, AVOCADO & RICOTTA
125 g (4½ oz) ricotta cheese
1 tablespoon basil pesto or Super Power
  Pesto (page 135)
75 g (2¾ oz) leg ham, finely chopped
½ large avocado, mashed

SMOKED SALMON
75 g (2¾ oz) cream cheese
1 teaspoon finely grated lemon zest
75 g (2¾ oz) smoked salmon, finely chopped
1 tablespoon finely chopped dill

CHICKEN WALDORF
75 g (2¾ oz) cooked chicken, finely chopped
½ celery stalk, finely chopped
½ small red apple, cored and grated
½ tablespoon crushed walnuts
½ teaspoon finely grated lemon zest
2 teaspoons garlic aioli

DUMPLINGS

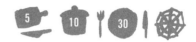

Making dumplings with your kids is a fun activity that will help them develop an appreciation of food.

250 g (9 oz) minced (ground) pork
2 tablespoons finely chopped chives
2 tablespoons finely chopped fresh coriander (cilantro) leaves
1 tablespoon finely grated fresh ginger
1 egg yolk
3 teaspoons salt-reduced soy sauce (GF if desired)
30 wonton wrappers

1 Mix the pork, chives, coriander, ginger, egg yolk and soy sauce together in a bowl.

2 Hold a wonton wrapper in one hand and put a heaped teaspoon of pork filling into the wrapper. Fold over and seal by wetting the edges with your fingertips dipped in water.

3 Line a steaming basket with baking paper and prick a couple of holes in the paper to allow steam to come through. Place the steaming basket over a wok of simmering water or large saucepan.

4 Steam dumplings in batches for about 10 minutes.

FOR TODDLER:

Serve with a little salt-reduced soy sauce for dipping.

ALL GROWN UP:

If you like a little heat, serve with some chilli oil.

SMART TIP

Coriander is a wonderful source of dietary fibre.

PUMPKIN & FETA ROLLS

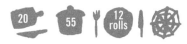

These vegetarian rolls offer a delicious alternative to the traditional sausage.

1 kg (2 lb 4 oz) butternut pumpkin (squash), peeled and diced
2 teaspoons dried sage
Olive oil, for cooking
Butter, for cooking
1 leek, finely chopped
2 garlic cloves, crushed
115 g (4 oz/1 cup) walnuts, crushed
200 g (7 oz) feta cheese, crumbled
2 sheets frozen puff pastry, thawed
1 egg, whisked

1 Preheat the oven to 180°C (350°F). Line a baking tray with baking paper and spread pumpkin over the tray. Toss with sage and olive oil, coating it evenly. Roast for 30 minutes or until the pumpkin starts to caramelise and develop a nice golden colour.

2 Meanwhile, melt a little butter in a heavy-based saucepan over medium heat and sauté the leek until softened. Add the garlic and walnuts and cook for a further minute.

3 Add the roasted pumpkin and feta to the leek mixture and mash it all together until smooth. Line two baking trays with baking paper. Cut each pastry sheet in half. Spread a quarter of the pumpkin mixture in a log along one long edge of each piece of pastry. Brush the opposite long edge with egg. Roll the pastry up to enclose the pumpkin mixture. Cut each roll into pieces.

4 Place the rolls, seam-side down, on the trays. Brush the tops of the rolls with egg. Bake for 25 minutes or until golden.

FOR TODDLER:

Great finger food for little hands. Ensure the walnuts are ground to avoid choking risk. For a nut-free school lunch, simply omit the walnuts.

ALL GROWN UP:

Great for a picnic play date.

SMART TIP

Walnuts are an incredible source of omega-3s, helping to aid healthy brain function. Try to build ground nuts into your child's daily diet.

SUSHI BALLS

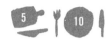

Fun for little fingers and a great way to build in some essential omega–3s.

2 tablespoons sushi seasoning
185 g (6½ oz/1 cup) cooked brown sushi rice
95 g (3¼ oz) tin tuna in olive oil, drained
1 hard-boiled egg, peeled
½ avocado
2 tablespoons Japanese-style mayonnaise
1 nori sheet
Salt-reduced soy sauce, to serve

1 Mix the sushi seasoning into the rice.

2 Mash the tuna, egg, avocado and mayonnaise together in a bowl.

3 With damp hands, form a clump of rice into a small cup and fill it with some tuna mixture. Take another clump of rice and close the ball. Roll in your hand to form a ball. Set aside and repeat with the remaining mixture and rice.

4 Cut fun shapes out of the nori and place on individual balls. Set for a few minutes in the fridge.

FOR TODDLER:

Put a little soy sauce in a bowl so they can have fun dipping. Vary the fillings to help build your child's taste preferences.

ALL GROWN UP:

Pickled ginger is a nice accompaniment.

SMART TIP
Seaweed (in the nori sheets) is a great source of choline, which plays an important role in nourishing brain cells.

BLUEBERRY FROZEN YOGHURT

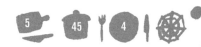

This is a better-for-you summer treat that kids just love.

4 tablespoons Greek-style
  yoghurt
2 handfuls of frozen
  blueberries
1 tablespoon maple syrup
  (more if you want it
  sweeter)
1 banana

1 Put all the ingredients in a blender and process until mixture has the texture of soft-serve ice cream.

2 Eat as it is or if you would like to make iceblocks (ice lollies, or popsicles) pour into moulds and insert a food-grade paddlepop stick into each mould. Freeze for 45 minutes before serving.

FOR TODDLER:

Serve as a soft-serve treat or make into iceblocks.

ALL GROWN UP:

Sprinkle with crushed pistachios for some crunch.

SMART TIP

Yoghurt and blueberries are a powerhouse combination. Yoghurt is a great probiotic for good digestive health and blueberries boost brain function.

FRUITY FINGERS

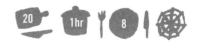

Nutritious, wholesome and perfect for when you are on the run.

245 g (8¾ oz/1½ cups) pitted dates, soaked in water for 1 hour
1 tablespoon natural vanilla extract
1 tablespoon coconut oil
25 g (1 oz/¼ cup) LSA meal (linseed, sunflower seed and almond)
2 tablespoons white chia seeds
100 g (3½ oz) desiccated coconut
235 g (8½ oz/1½ cups) dried apricots

1   Coarsely chop the dates and put in a food processor with the vanilla, coconut oil, LSA, chia seeds, half the desiccated coconut and 1 cup of the apricots.

2   Process for 2 minutes and transfer to a bowl. Finely chop the remaining apricots and add to the mixture.

3   Use your hands to shape small, finger-size portions and roll in the remaining coconut to coat.

4   Refrigerate for 1 hour before serving. Store in an airtight container in the fridge.

SMART TIP
Dates are rich in magnesium – a mineral known for its anti-inflammatory benefits.

MAC 'N' CHEESE CUPS

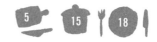

Macaroni cheese meets a muffin tin.

1 tablespoon butter, plus extra for greasing

155 g (5½ oz/1 cup) wholemeal macaroni

2 tablespoons wholemeal plain (all-purpose) flour (GF if desired)

125 ml (4 fl oz/½ cup) milk

25 g (1 oz/½ cup) spinach, finely chopped

1 spring onion (scallion), finely chopped

2 teaspoons fresh thyme leaves

150 g (5½ oz/1½ cups) grated cheddar cheese

1 Preheat the oven to 180°C (350°F). Lightly grease an 18-hole muffin tin with butter.

2 Cook the macaroni according to the packet instructions. Drain and transfer to a bowl.

3 Melt the butter in a small saucepan over low heat. Add the flour, stirring until it turns golden. Gradually stir in the milk until the mixture is smooth and simmering.

4 Remove from the heat. Add the cooked macaroni, spinach, spring onion, thyme and 100 g (3½ oz/ 1 cup) of the cheese.

5 Spoon into the muffin holes and top with the remaining cheese. Bake for 10–15 minutes until lightly browned.

FOR TODDLER:

Great for the lunchbox.

ALL GROWN UP:

Serve for lunch with a green salad.

SMART TIP

Spinach has extremely high nutritional value and is rich in antioxidants.

VEGGIE SLICE

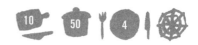

Nutrient dense and fun for little fingers.

5 eggs, lightly whisked
100 g (3½ oz) self-raising wholemeal flour (GF if desired)
1 teaspoon baking powder (GF if desired)
140 g (5 oz/1 cup) tinned sweet corn kernels
150 g (5½ oz/6 slices) bacon, chopped
1 large zucchini (courgette), grated
2 carrots, grated
1 red capsicum (pepper), chopped
1 brown onion, chopped
15 g (½ oz/½ cup) finely chopped fresh flat-leaf (Italian) parsley leaves
100 g (3½ oz1 cup) grated cheddar cheese

1 Preheat the oven to 180°C (350°F). Lightly grease a 20 x 30 cm (8 x 12 inch) baking tin or line with baking paper.

2 Combine the eggs, flour and baking powder in a bowl and whisk well. Stir in all the remaining ingredients.

3 Pour into the tin and bake for 50 minutes or until firm in the centre and golden brown.

FOR TODDLER:

Cut into fingers and serve with some Holy Guacamole (opposite).

ALL GROWN UP:

Serve with a green salad and balsamic dressing.

SMART TIP
Zucchini is high in fibre and a great source of plant-based omega–3s.

HOLY GUACAMOLE

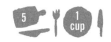

Toddlers love to dip. Offer this guacamole for a nutrient boost.

2 avocados
½ small red onion, finely chopped
Juice of 1 lime
1 tomato, seeds removed, finely chopped
15 g (½ oz/¼ cup) coarsely chopped coriander (cilantro) leaves

1 Mix together all of the ingredients in a food processor until smooth.

FOR TODDLER:

Toddlers love to dip, but this versatile guacamole can also be spread on toast or sandwiches or even stirred through cooked pasta.

ALL GROWN UP:

Season and add some jalapeños for a nice kick.

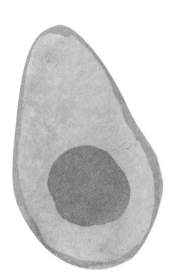

SMART TIP
Avocado is a great source of fibre. To keep avocado fresh and prevent it browning, put the avocado stone into the bowl until you're ready to use the mix.

SAVOURY SCROLLS

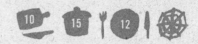

Savoury scrolls are always popular as a food-on-the-move option, but they aren't generally the most nutritious choice. By making these scrolls from scratch, you can increase their nutrient content.

250 g (8 oz) wholemeal self-raising flour

260 g (9¼ oz/1 cup) Greek-style yoghurt

3 tablespoons tomato paste (no-added-salt brand)

2 teaspoon dried Italian herbs

1 small handful of baby spinach leaves

¼ red capsicum (pepper), chopped

¼ red onion, thinly sliced

100 g (3½ oz) additive-free ham

150 g (5½ oz) tinned pineapple, finely chopped

100 g (3½ oz/1 cup) grated cheddar cheese

1 Preheat the oven to 200°C (400°F). Line a baking tray with baking paper.

2 Combine the flour and yoghurt in a large bowl and mix until they come together to form a ball of dough. If the dough is too sticky, add a little extra flour (about a tablespoon). Set the dough aside for 5 minutes to rest.

3 Transfer the dough to a lightly floured work surface and knead until it feels soft and stretchy.

4 Using a floured rolling pin, roll out to a 20 x 30 cm (8 x 12 inch) rectangle.

5 Spread the tomato paste over the dough, then top with the herbs, baby spinach, capsicum, red onion, ham, pineapple and grated cheese.

6 Roll the dough up from one short end as tightly as possible, so that you end up with a long sausage shape.

7 Slice into 12 pieces and arrange on the baking tray, cut side up, approximately 2.5 cm (1 inch) apart. Bake for 10–15 minutes until lightly golden.

Offer up different spreads and fillings for variety (see right).

ALL GROWN UP:

Great to put in a resealable plastic bag and take as a healthy snack item when on the move.

ALTERNATIVE FILLINGS:

Simply mix these ingredients together and spread over the dough.

ROASTED RED SPREAD
75 g (2¾ oz/½ cup) roasted capsicums
75 g (2¾ oz/½ cup) sun-dried tomatoes

GREEN GODDESS SPREAD
3 tablespoons Super Power Pesto (page 135)
    or ready-made basil pesto
1 small zucchini (courgette), grated

SMART TIP
Wholemeal flour provides iron, thiamine and niacin, as well as fibre.

PANCAKES FOR DINNER

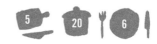

Have a little fun and serve some savoury pancakes for dinner. This delicious prawn okonomiyaki (Japanese pancake) will have your mini-me begging for more. You can swap the prawns for any protein.

225 g (8 oz/1½ cups) wholemeal plain (all-purpose) flour (GF if desired)
Rice bran oil, for frying
200 g (7 oz) raw prawns, peeled, chopped
6 eggs
75 g (2¾ oz/1 cup) shredded savoy cabbage
4 spring onions (scallions), finely chopped
200 g (7 oz/1 cup) tinned sweet corn kernels
Japanese-style mayonnaise, to serve
Kecap manis (sweet soy sauce), to serve

1 Put the flour in a bowl and gradually add 500 ml (17 fl oz/2 cups) of water, whisking to remove any lumps. Cover and put in the fridge for 30 minutes.

2 Meanwhile, heat a little rice bran oil in a small frying pan over medium heat and cook the prawn meat for 2 minutes or until opaque.

3 Remove the batter from the fridge and add the eggs. Whisk well. Stir in the prawns, cabbage, spring onion and corn.

4 Heat a little more oil in a small non-stick frying pan over low heat and pour one-third of a cup of batter into the pan. Cook for a few minutes until golden on the base and then flip over and cook the other side.

5 Serve with a drizzle of mayonnaise and kecap manis.

FOR TODDLER:

Make pikelet-size pancakes for finger-food fun.

ALL GROWN UP:

You can change the protein (try tuna, salmon or pork mince). Add some bonito flakes and pickled ginger for authentic flavour.

SMART TIP
Increasing your intake of plant-based foods such as cabbage can decrease the risk of lifestyle diseases.

FIVE-MINUTE FRIED RICE

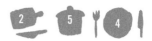

This healthy fried rice is a great meal to whip up at the last minute on a busy evening. You can make it a little more fancy with the addition of a protein such as prawns, chicken or bacon.

440 g (15½ oz) tinned pineapple pieces in natural juice
1 tablespoon rice bran oil
3 eggs, whisked
1 carrot, finely chopped
½ red capsicum (pepper)
80 g (2¾ oz/½ cup) unsalted cashew nuts, coarsely chopped (to avoid choking risk)
80 g (2¾ oz/½ cup) frozen peas and corn
2 garlic cloves, crushed
Family-size packet of microwave brown basmati rice, cooked according to packet directions
2 teaspoons curry powder
2 tablespoons salt-reduced soy sauce (GF if desired)
1 tablespoon fish sauce
30 g (1 oz/1 cup) fresh coriander (cilantro) leaves, to serve

1 Drain the pineapple, reserving 3 tablespoons juice.

2 Heat 2 teaspoons of the rice bran oil in a wok over high heat. Add the egg and swirl around to create a thin pancake. When egg is cooked through, remove from the wok and set aside.

3 Heat another 2 teaspoons of the oil in the wok and sauté the carrot, capsicum, cashews, pineapple, peas and corn until soft. Add the garlic and cook for a further minute. Add the rice and stir well. Add the curry powder, reserved pineapple juice, soy sauce and fish sauce. Add the egg, breaking it up with a spoon. Stir for 2 minutes and remove from the heat.

4 Serve with a scattering of fresh coriander leaves.

FOR TODDLER:

Ensure nuts are chopped up into small pieces to avoid choking risk.

ALL GROWN UP:

If you prefer a little more heat, add a bit more curry powder after serving your mini-me.

SMART TIP

Pineapple helps boost the immune system due to its high vitamin C content and antioxidants.

CHICKEN SCHNITZEL STRIPS

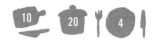

These chicken schnitzel strips are a nutritious alternative to the ready-made crumbed version.

150 g (5½ oz/1½ cups)
finely grated parmesan
cheese
150 g (5½ oz/1½ cups)
almond meal
10 g (½ oz/½ cup) flat-leaf
(Italian) parsley leaves,
finely chopped
2 eggs, lightly whisked
3 boneless, skinless chicken
breasts, sliced into strips
2 tablespoons olive oil
2 tablespoons butter
Lemon wedges, to serve

1 Mix together the parmesan, almond meal and chopped parsley in a flat bowl. Put the beaten egg in another bowl.

2 Dip the chicken strips into the egg and then into the parmesan mixture, coating well.

3 Heat the olive oil and butter in a frying pan over medium–high heat. Fry the chicken strips in batches until golden brown and cooked through.

FOR TODDLER:

Serve with a squeeze of lemon and mushy peas or Holy Guacamole (page 161).

ALL GROWN UP:

Season with salt and pepper and serve with peas and other vegetable side dishes.

SMART TIP

Olive oil is a cornerstone of the Mediterranean diet and very high in phenols – potent antioxidants, which are capable of lowering inflammation.

PASTA PERFECTION

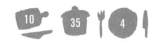

Fennel gives this dish a fabulous flavour and lentils provide a source of fibre for little tummies. This is a winning formula for the whole family.

2 tablespoons olive oil
1 brown onion, finely chopped
¼ red capsicum (pepper)
¼ small zucchini (courgette)
2 garlic cloves, crushed
1 teaspoon fennel seeds
1½ tablespoons tomato paste
500 g (1 lb 2 oz) good-quality pork sausages, casings removed
400 g (14 oz) tin lentils, rinsed
½ teaspoon chilli flakes
400 g (14 oz) tin chopped tomatoes
250 g (9 oz) small shell pasta (GF if desired)
Parmesan cheese, grated, to serve

1 Heat the olive oil in a large heavy-based frying pan. Sauté the onion, capsicum, zucchini and garlic until soft. Add the fennel seeds and stir for 1 minute.

2 Stir in the tomato paste, then add the sausage meat and stir to break up any lumps. Cook for 5 minutes until the meat is brown. Add the lentils, chilli flakes, tomatoes and 250 ml (9 fl oz/½ cup) of water. Lower the heat and simmer for 25 minutes.

3 Meanwhile, cook the pasta according to the packet directions and drain. Divide into bowls, top with the meat sauce and scatter with grated parmesan.

FOR TODDLER:

Don't be scared to add the chilli flakes – they only add a tiny bit of heat and help expand your toddler's taste preference.

ALL GROWN UP:

If you want to spice it up, add a little more chilli to the adult portions.

SMART TIP
Fennel can help relieve constipation. If your little one is suffering then increase their intake of fennel.

FRIDAY NIGHT PIZZA

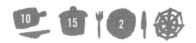

The traditional pizza dough has had a smart makeover with the addition of Greek yoghurt. Get the kids involved and let them come up with their own toppings.

260 g (9 oz/1 cup) Greek-style yoghurt
250 g (8 oz) self-raising wholemeal flour
Toppings (see opposite)

1 Preheat the oven to 180°C (350°F). Line a pizza tray with baking paper.

2 Mix the yoghurt and flour together and knead into a thick dough.

3 Divide the dough in half, lay on a floured surface and roll out with a rolling pin. Transfer to the pizza tray and add the sauce and toppings. Bake for about 15 minutes.

FOR TODDLER:

Toddlers love a sense of responsibility, so have them help choose their toppings.

ALL GROWN UP:

Get creative and offer a variety of toppings.

SMART TIP
Greek-style yoghurt is great for supporting a healthy gut microbiome.

TOPPINGS

SUPERPOWER PIZZA

Super Power Pesto (page 135)
150 g (5½ oz) raw prawns, peeled, deveined and chopped
1 tablespoon finely chopped red onion
100 g (3½ oz) haloumi cheese, grated
Lemon wedges, to serve

THE WORKS

3 tablespoons salt-reduced pizza sauce
2 teaspoons dried oregano
100 g (3½ oz) additive-free ham, chopped
80 g (2¾ oz) tinned pineapple pieces, drained
50 g (1¾ oz) olives, sliced
1 tablespoon finely chopped red onion
50 g (1¾ oz) marinated artichoke hearts
50 g (1¾ oz) green capsicum (pepper), chopped
50 g (1¾ oz) tomatoes, deseeded and chopped
50 g (1¾ oz) button mushrooms, chopped
100 g (3½ oz) parmesan or cheddar cheese, grated

VEGORAMA

70 g (2½ oz/¼ cup) Holy Guacamole (page 161)
200 g (7 oz) roasted pumpkin, thinly sliced
25 g (1 oz/½ cup) spinach leaves, chopped
3 tablespoons caramelised onion
3 tablespoons pine nuts, chopped for toddler
100 g (3½ oz) feta cheese, crumbled

BETTER-FOR-YOU BANGERS & MASH

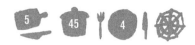

This is an Italian twist on the old favourite, bangers and mash. Most fussy eaters will eat sausages and we have added some smart ingredients to make this a more nutritious option for your family. It will be a favourite in no time and is particularly lovely with Supercharged Mash (page 49).

2 tablespoons olive oil
6–8 good-quality sausages
½ red capsicum (pepper), finely chopped
1 onion, finely chopped
1 celery stalk, finely chopped
1 carrot, peeled and finely chopped
1 teaspoon fennel seeds
1 teaspoon dried Italian herbs
400 g (14 oz) tinned four-bean mix, rinsed
125 ml (4 fl oz/½ cup) salt-reduced beef stock (GF if desired)
80 g (2¾ oz/½ cup) frozen peas and corn
2 tablespoons tomato paste
400 g (14 oz) tin chopped tomatoes
Honey, maple syrup or rice malt syrup, to sweeten

1 Heat half the olive oil in a heavy-based saucepan and cook the sausages until just browned. Remove from the pan and set aside. Add the remaining oil to the pan and cook the capsicum, onion, celery and carrot until softened. Add the fennel seeds and Italian herbs and stir until fragrant.

2 Cut each sausage into 6–7 small chunks with kitchen scissors. Put the sausage, beans, stock, peas and corn, tomato paste and tomatoes into the pan. Stir well and bring to a very gentle simmer over low heat. Cover and gently simmer for 20 minutes. Add a little honey or other sweetener to cut through the bitterness.

FOR TODDLER:

Sausages can be a choking risk if they are not cut into small bite-size pieces and remove any skin.

ALL GROWN UP:

Season well or kick it up a notch with some hot sauce.

SMART TIP
Beans are a powerhouse of nutrients, including antioxidants, vitamins and minerals. They are a staple of the Mediterranean diet and a great source of fibre.

BAKED CARBONARA

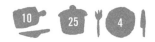

Sometimes you just need a comforting cheesy dish and this baked carbonara does the trick, but with the addition of a few nutritious twists.

1 tablespoon butter
1 brown onion, finely chopped
150 g (5½ oz) asparagus, finely chopped
150 g (5½ oz) pancetta or bacon, finely chopped
90 g (3¼ oz/1 cup) finely chopped mushrooms
2 garlic cloves, crushed
250 g (9 oz) dried bowtie pasta (GF if desired)
2 large egg yolks
60 ml (2 fl oz/¼ cup) salt-reduced vegetable stock (GF if desired)
150 ml 5 fl oz) pure (35% fat) cream
100 g (3½ oz/1 cup) finely grated parmesan cheese
60 g (2¼ oz/1 cup) fresh wholemeal breadcrumbs (GF if desired)
2 tablespoons chopped fresh flat-leaf (Italian) parsley leaves
30 g (1 oz/¼ cup) crushed walnuts
1 tablespoon olive oil
100 g (3½ oz/¾ cup) frozen minted peas
Lemon, to serve

1 Preheat the oven to 200°C (400°F). Put a saucepan of water on the stove to boil.

2 Heat the butter in a frying pan over medium heat and fry the onion, asparagus, pancetta and mushrooms until softened. Add the garlic and continue to fry for 1 minute more. Set aside.

3 Cook the pasta in the saucepan of boiling water until tender but not completely cooked through. Drain and immediately stir in the egg yolks.

4 Combine the pasta with the asparagus mixture, vegetable stock, cream and half of the parmesan. Pour into an ovenproof dish.

5 Mix together the remaining parmesan, breadcrumbs, parsley, walnuts and olive oil. Scatter the crumb mixture over the pasta and bake for 15 minutes.

6 Meanwhile, cook the peas. Stir the peas into the carbonara and serve with a squeeze of lemon.

FOR TODDLER:

Many toddlers have a taste for lemon and it helps to cut through the creaminess here.

ALL GROWN UP:

Season with pepper.

SMART TIP

Walnuts contain neuroprotective compounds, including vitamin E, folate, omega–3 fats and antioxidants.

INDEX

NOTES

1. Du Toit G, Katz Y, Sasieni P, Mesher D, Maleki SJ, Fisher HR, Fox AT, Turcanu V, Amir T, Zadik-Mnuhin G, Cohen A, Livne I, Lack G *Early consumption of peanuts in infancy is associated with a low prevalence of peanut allergy.* J Allergy Clin Immunol. 2008 Nov;122(5):984-91.

2. Nyaradi A, Jianghong L, Foster JK, Oddy W (2015) *Good-quality diet in the early years may have a positive effect on academic achievement.* Acta Paediatrica 105(5).

3. Nyaradi A, Oddy WH, Hickling S, Li J, Foster JK (2015) *The relationship between nutrition in infancy and cognitive performance during adolescence.* Front Nutr. 2:2.

4. Gale CR, Martyn CN, Marriott LD, Limond J, Crozier S, Inskip HM, et al (2009) *Dietary patterns in infancy and cognitive and neuropsychological function in childhood.* J Child Psychol Psychiatry 50, 816–23.

5. Smithers LG, Golley RK, Mittinty MN, Brazionis L, Northstone K, Emmett P, et al (2012) *Dietary patterns at 6,15 and 24 months of age are associated with IQ at 8 years of age.* Eur. J Epidemiol. 27, 525–35.

Published in 2018 by Murdoch Books, an imprint of Allen & Unwin

Murdoch Books Australia
83 Alexander Street
Crows Nest NSW 2065
Phone: +61 (0)2 8425 0100
murdochbooks.com.au
info@murdochbooks.com.au

Murdoch Books UK
Ormond House, 26–27 Boswell Street,
London, WC1N 3JZ
Phone: +44 (0) 20 8785 5995
murdochbooks.co.uk
info@murdochbooks.co.uk

For Corporate Orders & Custom Publishing contact our business development team at
salesenquiries@murdochbooks.com.au

Publisher: Jane Morrow
Editorial Manager: Jane Price
Design Manager: Hugh Ford
Designer and Illustrator: Arielle Gamble
Editor: Melody Lord
Production Manager: Lou Playfair

ISBN 978 1 76063 174 1 Australia
ISBN 978 1 76063 444 5 UK

A cataloguing-in-publication entry is available from the catalogue of
the National Library of Australia at nla.gov.au
A catalogue record for this book is available from the British Library

Printed and bound by Leo Paper Group, China

DISCLAIMER: The content presented in this book is meant for inspiration and informational purposes
only. The purchaser of this book understands that the author is not a medical professional, and the
information contained within this book is not intended to replace medical advice or meant to be
relied upon to treat, cure or prevent any disease, illness or medical condition. It is understood that
you will seek full medical clearance by a licensed physician before making any changes mentioned
in this book. The author and publisher claim no responsibility to any person or entity for any liability,
loss or damage caused or alleged to be caused directly or indirectly as a result of the use, application
or interpretation of the material in this book.

OVEN GUIDE: You may find cooking times vary depending on the oven you are using. For fan-forced
ovens, as a general rule, set the oven temperature to 20°C (70°F) lower than indicated in the recipe.

MEASURES GUIDE: We have used 20 ml (4 teaspoon) tablespoon measures. If you are using a
15 ml (3 teaspoon) tablespoon add an extra teaspoon of the ingredient for each tablespoon specified.